HOSPICE
A Photographic Inquiry

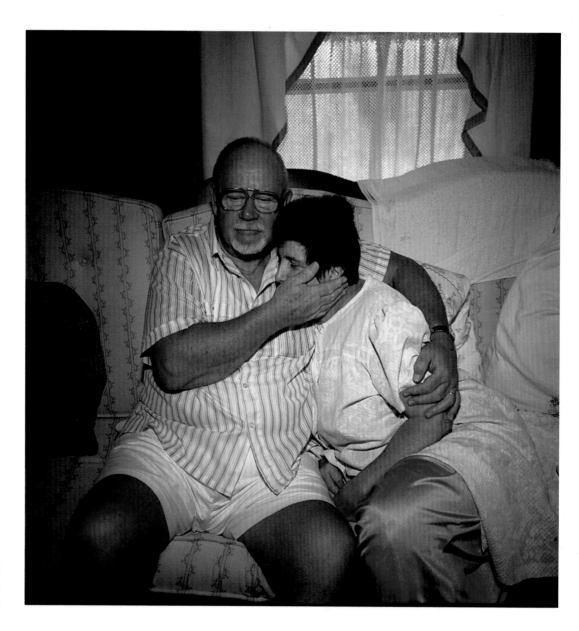

Nan Goldin
Grace and Carl at Home,
Riverhead, New York, 1995

HOSPICE
A Photographic Inquiry

Photographs by

JIM GOLDBERG

NAN GOLDIN

SALLY MANN

JACK RADCLIFFE

KATHY VARGAS

Edited by
Dena Andre, Philip Brookman,
and Jane Livingston

With essays by
Marilyn Webb and Jane Livingston

Interviews by
Philip Brookman

Stills from a film by
Susan Froemke, Deborah Dickson,
and Albert Maysles

A Bulfinch Press Book
Little, Brown and Company
Boston   New York   Toronto   London
In association with the Corcoran Gallery of Art
and the National Hospice Foundation

Major funding for *Hospice: A Photographic Inquiry* has been provided by **WARNER LAMBERT**, a pharmaceutical and consumer products company, as part of its ongoing commitment to supporting hospice care in the United States and around the world. The exhibition has also been supported by a generous gift from The Project on Death in America, funded by the Open Society Institute, a nonprofit foundation that supports the development of open societies worldwide. Additional support has been received from the National Endowment for the Arts, The Prudential Foundation, the Glen Eagles Foundation, and Learning Design Associates, Inc.

First Edition

Book design by Caroline Rowntree

Library of Congress Cataloging-in-Publication Data
Hospice : a photographic inquiry / Corcoran Gallery of Art and National Hospice Foundation; photographs by Jim Goldberg, Nan Goldin, Sally Mann, Jack Radcliffe, Kathy Vargas; edited by Dena Andre, Philip Brookman, and Jane Livingston; with essays by Marilyn Webb and Jane Livingston. — 1st ed.
    p. cm.
    Includes bibliographical references (p.).
    ISBN 0-8212-2259-7 — ISBN 0-8212-2260-0 (pbk.)
    1. Hospices — United States — Pictorial works — Exhibitions. 2. Hospice care — United States — Pictorial works — Exhibitions. 3. Hospice care — Miscellanea. I. Corcoran Gallery of Art. II. National Hospice Foundation. III. Andre, Dena. IV. Brookman, Philip. V. Livingston, Jane.
    RA1000.3.H67   1996
    362.1'75 — dc20   95-30088

Bulfinch Press is an imprint and trademark of Little, Brown and Company
Published simultaneously in Canada by Little, Brown & Company (Canada) Limited
Printed in the United States of America

Hospice: A Photographic Inquiry exhibition tour:
The Corcoran Gallery of Art, Washington, D.C., March 9–May 5, 1996. **Wexner Center for the Arts,** The Ohio State University, Columbus, Ohio, May 17–August 4, 1996. **Chicago Cultural Center,** Chicago, Illinois, September 21–November 17, 1996. **The Morris Museum,** Morristown, New Jersey, January 5–February 23, 1997. **San Diego Museum of Art,** San Diego, California, June 7–July 20, 1997. **Telfair Academy of Arts and Sciences,** Savannah, Georgia, August 19–October 26, 1997. **Norton Gallery and School of Art,** West Palm Beach, Florida, November 15, 1997–January 11, 1998. **Marjorie Barrick Museum of Natural History,** University of Nevada, Las Vegas, Nevada, February 1–April 30, 1998. **Phoenix Art Museum,** Phoenix, Arizona, May 15–July 26, 1998. **David Winton Bell Gallery,** Brown University, Providence, Rhode Island, October 24–November 29, 1998. **New Orleans Museum of Art,** New Orleans, Louisiana, February 20–April 18, 1999. **Frederick R. Weisman Art Museum,** University of Minnesota, Minneapolis, Minnesota, April 14–June 18, 2000. **Portland Art Museum,** Portland, Oregon, dates to be announced.

CONTENTS

1   Preface by Zachary P. Morfogen

2   Introduction by David C. Levy

5   "Death and Dying in America" by Marilyn Webb

13   "Hospice: A Photographic Inquiry" by Jane Livingston

        Portfolios, with interviews by Philip Brookman

        24   JIM GOLDBERG

        52   NAN GOLDIN

        76   SALLY MANN

        106   JACK RADCLIFFE

        130   KATHY VARGAS

156   "Hospice on Film: Three Stories" by Philip Brookman

160   "Hospice Care Today" by John J. Mahoney

162   Hospice: Bibliography

164   Acknowledgments

166   Photographers: Biographical Information

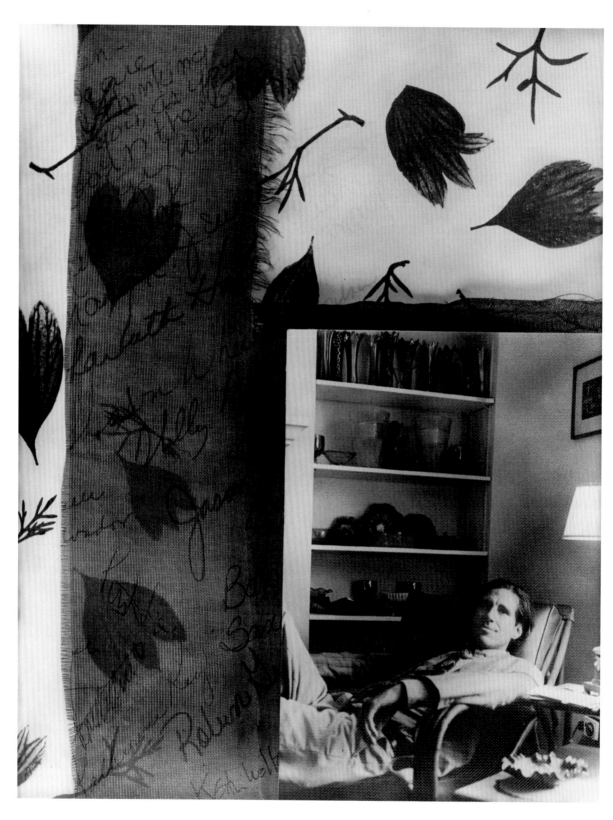

Kathy Vargas
Don and Bill:
Don in His Apartment, 1994

PREFACE

*I*n the founding days of the National Hospice Organization, the spirit that encouraged us was, "fresh and green are the meadows where He gives me rest." With that inspiration, the hospice concept has gained rapid acceptance since the first U.S. hospice opened in New Haven, Connecticut, in 1974. Last year more than 340,000 patients received hospice care, and there were over 2,000 hospices in America caring not only for cancer patients and their families but also for those in the terminal stage of AIDS, Alzheimer's, and other diseases.

In 1978, when the National Hospice Organization was launched, *Time* magazine ran an article headlined "A Better Way of Dying: *Hospices help ease the pain and fear of the terminally ill.*" *Time* concluded, "As the U.S. begins to cope more directly with the once taboo subject of death, the hospice idea is likely to spread even farther and faster." As the first chairman of NHO, I was quoted: "Death has finally come out of the closet." During that *Time* interview two questions were raised that continue to come up whenever hospice is discussed: "What is hospice?" and "Why are you involved?"

Personally and professionally I have always been committed to the arts. My wife, an active hospital volunteer, suggested that she become involved in the arts and I, with health care. That led me to the presidency of Riverside Hospital in Boonton, New Jersey, and from there I visited St. Christopher's Hospice in London and met Dame Cicely Saunders, founder of the modern hospice movement. Her conviction — "*You matter because of who you are. You matter to the last moment of your life, and we will do all we can not only to help you die peacefully, but also to live until you die.*" — inspired the development of Riverside Hospice, the first freestanding hospice in America. We were guided by Hospice Inc. in New Haven, and together we organized the 2nd National Hospice Symposium, which led to the founding of the National Hospice Organization.

Five years ago, the dynamic leaders and members of NHO determined the need for the National Hospice Foundation, to broaden America's understanding of hospice through research and education and to better answer the question, "What is hospice?" The foundation first funded a Gallup Poll, which revealed that a clear majority of Americans want to be cared for and die at home, but that most are unaware that hospice offers such an opportunity.

The foundation determined that organizing *Hospice: A Photographic Inquiry* as a major public outreach project was appropriate to broaden America's understanding of hospice through the personal involvement and insights of some of the country's most sensitive artists. Throughout history, the arts have had a dramatic impact on social issues and change. Our partnership with the Corcoran Gallery of Art to organize this exhibition, and with our colleagues at HBO and Bulfinch Press, is personally gratifying.

The dedication of the founders, members, staff, directors, trustees, governors, volunteers, and sponsors that have brought hospice care to this moment of "fresh and green" opportunity is celebrated as we proceed with our mission of expanding America's vision for end-of-life care.

Zachary P. Morfogen
Chairman
National Hospice Foundation

INTRODUCTION

My generation of Americans never learned to cope very well with death. Our parents did better because they grew up in a world that recognized dying as part of living. Perhaps they were closer, in what seems to have been a simpler time, to the natural order of things. What is certain is that, for them, it was common to lose friends or loved ones by the age of puberty. Dying and grieving were part of community life — whether in city neighborhoods, small towns, or rural farmlands. Mostly people died at home, where their families closed ranks in mutual support, helping both the dying and themselves to face the unknowable.

Most of us who grew up in the aura of scientific and technological faith that has marked postwar America have had a different experience. Often we have known our parents well into our own middle age. Few of us as children experienced the death of a friend. Pneumonia, polio, smallpox, and TB — fatal and commonplace in our parents' generation — have been all but banished from ours; and, most important, we have been protected, if not insulated, from the dying. Indeed, to us, the very idea of death is only marginally discussable. Rather than accept and deal with this inevitable right of passage, midcentury, middle-class America made it the ultimate taboo. Four years ago Marilyn Webb aptly wrote that we kept death "locked behind hospital doors. . . ." As is the usual case with incarceration, in so doing we also reduced our chances of coming to terms with the prisoner.

Ironically, at a moment in history when technology in every discipline is expanding exponentially, we are moving back toward our parents' gentler understanding of death — accepting it with a new humanism as an integral, dignified part of our life process and, importantly, bringing the dying back into our homes. The hospice movement has been a crucial component of this change.

A central theme of hospice is the belief that the terminally ill should be relieved of pain and that, wherever possible, the dying should have the dignity and support of home and family. That hospice has been successful in bringing both these messages and the techniques that support them to millions of families over a relatively short period of time is, perhaps, not surprising when we consider how resonant a human chord is struck by such basic precepts.

The purpose of this exhibition, therefore, is to expand our understanding of the power and importance of hospice, seeing it through the perspective of the artist's eye. In choosing photography as our medium, we selected a vehicle that many associate instinctively with journalism and documentation. But reportage is not our purpose. Rather, we wish to share artistic insights born of an immersion into hospice and the people it serves — the dying and their families. The sharing that comes to us through the work of the gifted photographers who accepted this creative challenge achieves a level of communication and meaning that only art makes possible. Despite its diversity of approach, their work consistently rises above physical distress and imminent tragedy to show us the humanity and spirit embedded in this ultimate journey of life, and in the ordinary people who are its subject.

This exhibition tells us that while hospice may not be an answer for all the dying, it is of immeasurable help to many who would otherwise be in agony, despair, and need. We hope it will be as revealing and helpful to its audience as it has been to its creators.

Hospice: A Photographic Inquiry concludes three years of work by the Corcoran's curator of photography and media arts, Philip Brookman, by its guest co-curators, the noted photographic scholar Jane Livingston, her associate Dena Andre, and by their staffs. They and the artists whom they commissioned to explore this difficult and emotionally treacherous subject have, together, shared an odyssey through the most profound of human experiences. The important work they have accomplished would not have been possible if others had not believed with us that humanity would be richer for the unique understanding their combined vision would achieve. Our deepest thanks, therefore, go to the Warner-Lambert Company; The Project on Death in America, a program of the Open Society Institute; the National Endowment for the Arts; The Prudential Foundation; the Glen Eagles Foundation; the National Hospice Foundation; and Learning Design Associates, Inc., whose generous support made this exhibition a reality.

David C. Levy
President and Director
The Corcoran Gallery of Art

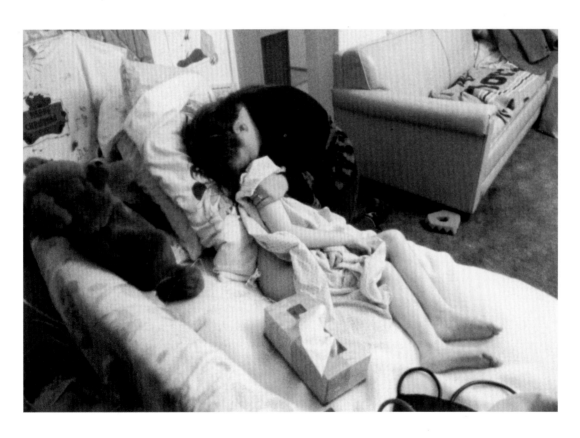

Susan Froemke, Deborah Dickson, and Albert Maysles
Michael Merseal, Jr., with his mother, Debra Woodward, Missoula, Montana, 1995

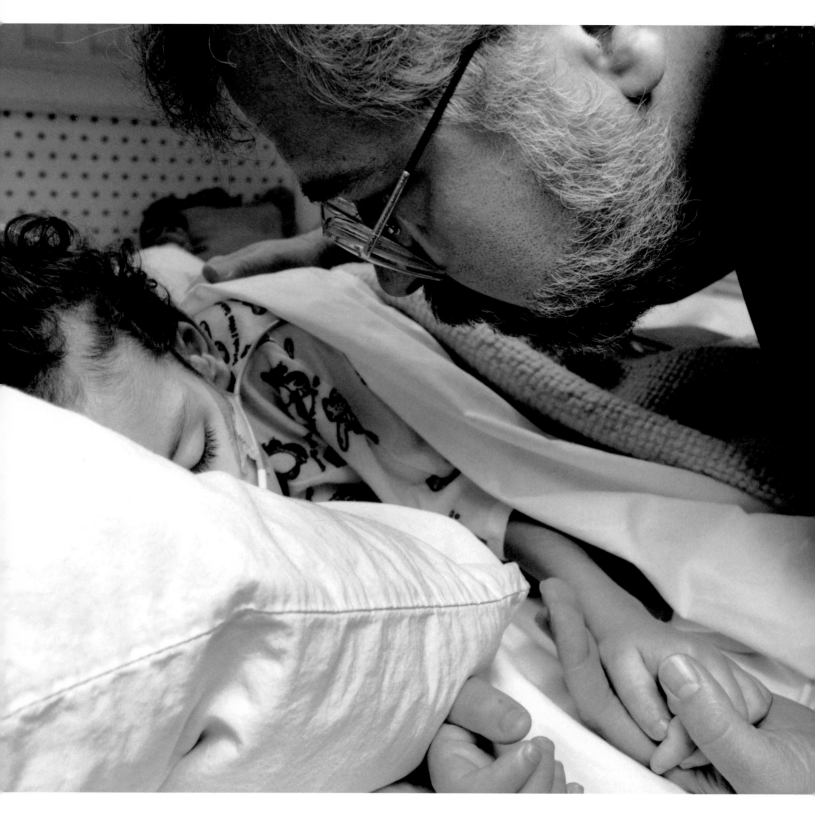

Jack Radcliffe
Boo Boo, March 26, 1993

DEATH AND DYING IN AMERICA
BY MARILYN WEBB

*I*t's April 23, 1992. At Cabrini Hospice's in-patient unit in Manhattan, fifty-nine-year-old Audrey Hill is dying. She has lost sixty pounds and is lying in bed, cheeks caved in, great gaps in her mouth where caps have fallen off. She is clutching a soft stuffed rabbit.

When I walk in and am introduced, Audrey looks up from her pillow and smiles with the most incredibly warm eyes. She sticks out her hand and says, graciously, "Hello, I'm Audrey." Her breathing stops often, for great lengths of time, making it seem as if there will be no more breaths. Then, casually, she takes another.

Sometimes Audrey stares at nothing. Then she comes back. And smiles. She says that when she's "away" it's like sleeping. When she comes back, after one her of lapses, she takes my hand and strokes it, as if to calm me and says, "Tell me about your loves." She is grateful for very small things — sips of water from a cup held by more steady hands, a pillow fluffed, someone to hold her hand — so full of compassion and humor.

Audrey didn't die that April day, but in June. By then she had taught me something profound, that as awful as it is to lose someone you love, death isn't necessarily terrifying. And that lesson transformed anything I'd thought before about death and dying. I realized that it was hospice that had made all the difference.

Audrey's story, the story that brought her to Cabrini, illustrates what makes hospice so special. Before she became ill, Audrey was a workaholic, a career woman raising two now-adult children, working eighteen-hour days as the founding president of a travel company. Her husband had died of cancer ten years before. She herself was diagnosed with inoperable cervical cancer in January of 1991. By February she was given only forty days to live.

Audrey's chances of survival were small, so she made the crucial decision that she'd rather have help with her pain than prolong her illness with torturous treatments. She called Cabrini Hospice. Her twenty-eight-year-old son, Jonathan, got a larger apartment so she could move in with him, and Cabrini sent home-care aides, nurses, a doctor, pain medications, a hospital bed, plus social workers and music and art therapists to help. But Audrey didn't die, as doctors expected.

"She's said that except for the fact that she's dying," Jonathan says, "this has been the most terrific time of her life." With her pain controlled, she was able to continue working until June. After she stopped, she began cooking, doing needlepoint, learning to play the guitar — things she never had time for. She also held late-night salons with friends, having philosophical discussions on dying. But her health steadily declined; she had a stroke, she broke her hip, she entered a roller-coaster time of last breaths and revivals. Something, no one could figure out what, was making Audrey hang on.

On that day I first met her, I was accompanying Sister Loretta Palamara — Cabrini's spiritual counselor, known in hospice circles to be especially gifted in helping people die peaceful deaths — on her rounds. When someone as sick as Audrey still resists death, Sister Loretta tells me, it's often because of some unfinished business. They might be waiting for the birth of a grandchild or to see the wedding gown of a child about to be married, or to hear something as simple as a last *I love you* or *I forgive you* or *I'm sorry.* "Usually, if you find the right thing, people will go on the spot," she says. "You have to stay open to find out what that thing is. If you're filled with judgments, you won't find anything. But if your heart is open, you will."

Yet Sister Loretta had something more to tell me. When she was twenty-five, she was hit by lightning as she was trying to close a window in her convent for an elderly nun. In 1969, when she was thirty-six,

Sister Loretta nearly died from an embolism that doctors said was caused by complications from the lightning. Lying in her hospital bed, she had a classic near-death experience, feeling herself traveling through a tunnel, experiencing a deep sense of peace, seeing a bright light emanating intense love, and finding the elderly nun, who had since died, coming to greet her, telling her to go back, she had a mission to do, that it wasn't yet her time. Only later did Sister Loretta realize that her mission must be to work with the dying. She uses that experience now as her guide, as her way of speaking the spiritual language of death so all people can hear, no matter what their religious or secular convictions. And in the end, that may have been what helped Audrey.

By the time she died — almost two months after I first met her — Audrey was back home, spending her days in a hospital bed in her son's living room. Each day, while Jonathan went to work, her daughter, Margaret, twenty-six, and Margaret's two children came over. Friends came by, and in the evenings there would be the salon. Audrey lay in the center of it, beaming. Then something began to change. She started sleeping more. When she awoke, she'd say she was getting ready to go on a journey, packing her bags, getting her ticket, things she knew she needed from the travel business. Then she said the words that revealed what had been keeping her from dying. Audrey told everyone she was waiting for her dead husband to come and get her.

Soon she grew serene. She smiled in her sleep. She held Jonathan's hand. She told Margaret and her grandchildren she loved them. She'd listen to music and talk to friends, but she was waiting. Listening. Looking at the ceiling or the wall. Then one day she announced that her husband had come, that he was here, now, in the living room with her. She grew enormously calm. She began talking to him as if he were sitting on the couch, standing near. After a while, she decided to say good-bye.

A few mornings later, while she and a friend were watching a movie on TV, Audrey just quietly died. Sister Loretta says she'd chosen a time when it was easier to leave than if her whole family was standing by. "I feel like I'm a midwife, like I'm pushing new life. But instead of saying, 'Push, push, push,' I'm always saying, 'Go toward the light. Look for your relatives and friends.'" That's probably just what Audrey did.

*T*he way Audrey died is not how we normally think of death. Nor is her quiet passage the experience of those who spend their final days hospitalized. There were no tubes, no last-minute surgeries, no IVs, no CPR, no respirators. But there also wasn't any panic or fear. In a way, Sister Loretta was right: it *was* very much like a birthing.

Over the next three years, I crisscrossed the country, trying to see if Audrey's experience was common. I visited hospitals, nursing homes, and hospices. I talked with doctors, psychologists, social workers, and theologians. I spent time with dying patients and their families. I talked with the kinds of people you will see in this exhibition, people from rural towns in Virginia, cities in Texas or Pennsylvania or Florida. What I found is that, as a nation, Americans are spontaneously, at the grassroots level, creating a new way to prepare for death. And hospice is at the center of it.

A movement has emerged that has begun to explore *natural dying*, much as the Lamaze movement explored natural childbirth three decades ago. This is a movement that rests on a revolution in medicine, a sea change in medical technology and a revamping of end-of-life law. It's a movement that's spiritual, but it's not traditionally religious. Its proponents are trying to help those they love die the deaths they choose — dignified deaths when the prognoses are terminal and further treatments are of question-able value. Like natural childbirth, *natural dying* is returning death to the intimacy of American families and homes. But just as medical advances — like pain medications and fetal monitors — have been incorporated into natural childbirth, modern medications can now manage pain or other uncomfortable symptoms at death. And new laws have given us unprecedented ability to say no to unwanted treatments.

Today there are 2,100 hospices nationwide. They care for 14 percent of us as we die, some 340,000 people a year — about 35 percent of all cancer and AIDS deaths, and a smaller percentage of those who die of other illnesses. Some hospices have in-patient units in hospitals, like Cabrini's; others have residential centers for those with no one able to stay home with them. But most hospices primarily offer help to families who want to care for a loved one at home.

To understand what led us to this new approach to dying, it's helpful to look back at the extraor-dinary medical advances of the past two hundred years, and particularly at the pace of these advances just since World War II, during the maturing of the baby-boom generation.

At the turn of the century, most Americans died at home from infectious or parasitic diseases — illnesses like typhoid, yellow fever, or cholera; wound infections; or complications of childbirth — whose course from onset to death was relatively swift. Except for tuberculosis, death generally took about a week, maybe ten days at most. The average life expectancy was only fifty years. But by 1900 improvements in anesthesia had already started making more sophisticated surgery possible. Bacteria and viruses began to be isolated as the causes of disease. Public health measures were being put in place to curb the spread of epidemics like cholera, and vaccines against yellow fever and typhoid were well on the way. In 1908 the age of chemical therapy truly began, when scientist Paul Ehrlich won the Nobel Prize for discovering that certain chemicals could kill bacteria. In the 1940s antibiotics finally appeared — first sulfonamides, which turned out to have dangerous side effects, and shortly thereafter, the miracle drug penicillin.

When the front-runners of the baby-boom generation were born, medicine was entering an unprecedented age, an age when illnesses could truly be prevented, treated, and cured. In the 1950s polio was eradicated within one year. Vaccines practically eliminated childhood diseases like measles and German measles. A cure for tuberculosis nearly banished that dreaded disease. Life expectancy moved up to the age of seventy. Baby boomers became the first generation to grow up not surrounded by early deaths from anything other than war. And they grew up believing that medicine could cure anything.

Today, Americans no longer die swiftly, as they did at the turn of the century. Countless medical miracles such as kidney dialysis have become everyday procedures; unheard-of operations like bypass sur-gery and organ transplants are commonplace. Advanced methods of diagnosis — CAT scans, MRIs, mam-mograms, sonograms, angiograms — abound. These have all brought about a revolution in how we die. We are surviving infections that once killed us quickly, only to live long enough for the body to slowly wear out. Now our major killers are the degenerative diseases: heart disease, cancer, stroke or cardio-vascular disease, Alzheimer's, and lung disease. But while medical advances have allowed lives that might have been lost to be saved, they have also meant that the time we spend chronically ill has grown longer, even now with modern diseases like AIDS.

It is apparent that medicine's success has been truly miraculous. Yet it is also now apparent that it has brought with it a culture of aggressive treatment. Starting in the 1970s, it seems, the goals of medicine dangerously shifted from maintaining health and warding off suffering to the battle to cure and ward off death by any means, no matter what the financial, physical, or emotional cost for patients or families. It was in the 1970s that people began to question how the medical profession was handling death and dying. This climate of concern allowed for the birth of American hospice.

*T*he history of hospice in America begins not on American shores but in England. It originated in the work of an Englishwoman named Cicely Saunders, a nursing student during World War II who saw much suffering and death. She realized that what mattered most at the end of life seemed to be pain control and dignity in dying. She also saw two kinds of pain: physical pain, and the psychological and spiritual pain of death itself. By the time she returned from the war, Saunders already understood what she wanted to do with that knowledge.

First she got a degree in social work; next she got a degree in medicine. Then she began working in hospices around London, which at the time were places where nuns took care of the dying — rather like those run by Mother Teresa in India. Hospices have, in fact, existed since medieval times, but until recently they did not just care for the dying. They were way stations for travelers, places for the weary to recover, the pregnant to give birth, and the ill to either get well or die. They were resting places, usually run by a religious order.

Dr. Saunders wanted to combine this idea of caregiving with the best of modern medicine, and particularly with the best pain medication she could find. She discovered a blend of heroin or morphine, cocaine, alcohol, and antinausea medication, named "Brompton Cocktail" after the British hospital that created it; she would become a pioneer in giving it in steady doses round the clock, so pain never had a chance to peak.

In 1967 Dr. Saunders began her own hospice near London — St. Christopher's, housed in a sprawling old home surrounded by gardens and stone walls. It has a chapel, a child-care center, a room for afternoon tea, a bar for night discussions, and space where patients can spend time with their families and friends. But it provides care only for the dying.

St. Christopher's first goal was to make sure patients got their pain — or other uncomfortable symptoms — under control. Then it went on to its next mission — to help the terminally ill do their own work of dying. That, in Dr. Saunders's view, means coming to terms with "who you are, what the world is about, and what your place in it somehow is — the search for meaning." She believes a good hospice provides an environment where people can find a wider view of life — through art, music, love, relationships, family, beauty, or religion.

At the same time that Dr. Saunders was launching St. Christopher's in England, Elisabeth Kübler-Ross, a Swiss physician then at the University of Chicago, was beginning to shape insights that would forever change our thinking about death. Dr. Kübler-Ross happened to be among the first to see inside a German concentration camp soon after it was opened, a camp where nearly a million children had died. Scratched on the walls with tiny fingernails, next to the little bunk beds, besides messages of love to mommies and daddies, were hundreds and hundreds of butterflies. She wondered a long time what those butterflies meant. After years of treating dying patients herself, she began to understand and to teach what she had learned. In 1969 she published her landmark book, *On Death and Dying*. Dying is a process, Dr. Kübler-Ross says, and at death there is a metamorphosis of the human spirit — much like a butterfly breaking free of its cocoon. In her book she describes in detail the psychological process of dying, and the symbolic and spiritual thinking that dying patients — like Audrey — inevitably use.

The pioneering thinking of these two women, Drs. Saunders and Kübler-Ross, coalesced in the work of an American nurse, Florence Wald, who created the very first hospice in America.

Wald had started working in the 1940s as a young nurse, and by the mid-1960s she was dean at Yale University's school of nursing. It was part of Yale–New Haven Medical Center, an institution on the forefront of high-tech advances. Wald had watched as medicine moved from a focus on people, as she put it, to a focus on their diseases. This was of particular concern to her because of her responsibility to train future generations of nurses. It disturbed her deeply that death was not even talked about, and that the impact of treatment itself on patients and families was not, either. "Communication was lacking between caregivers and patients," she says, "and the way decisions were made excluded patients."

Wald sought new solutions in the work of both Saunders and Kübler-Ross. She brought them together to speak at Yale. The turning point came in 1968, when she chose to spend her vacation working at St. Christopher's, which had opened just the year before. Wald rented a house in London, taking her whole family with her, in order to spend a month nursing the dying, something she hadn't done in years. Her days with Saunders at St. Christopher's left her ecstatic. Back in New Haven, she couldn't stop talking about it, sharing her enthusiasm with friends and colleagues, among them doctors and a minister, often over her own kitchen table in Connecticut. It was in that state, in Branford, in 1974 that the first American hospice was born. Wald resigned as dean of the school of nursing to focus solely on forming this hospice and reshaping the care of the dying.

The Connecticut Hospice began by offering home care. Eventually, Wald and her co-founders built an in-patient residence. But as the hospice movement has grown in America, it has commonly emphasized — as Wald's hospice does — care and medical support in patients' homes rather than care in a residential facility.

Here, as abroad, hospice care always puts the focus on humane dying. And the secret of humane dying is assuaging pain, so that the patient's real work, the psychological work of dying, can go on. Today, medications are far more sophisticated than they were when hospice began: modern narcotics, including morphine, are given in liquid form; there are sustained-release capsules, skin patches, patient-controlled pumps, IVs, and high-tech surgical treatments. Today, there is a better understanding about various kinds of pain and how to deliver medications to specific pain sites. Myths persist about addiction or overdosing, but hospice has been in the forefront of trying to break them. Great strides have been made in just the past few years to ensure adequate treatment of serious pain, which, properly done, requires *as much medication as patients themselves feel they need to take*.

In a hospice setting, once pain is under control it is the job of the hospice workers to move on to the psychological and spiritual dimensions. And that remains what Dr. Saunders described as the work of dying. While she relied heavily on the Church of England, once hospice came to America it became infused with a larger spirituality — one that can include a belief such as Kübler-Ross's or Sister Loretta's rather than an adherence to just one particular religion. America is a diverse nation, and good hospices here seem to be able to assist in life closure, whatever that might mean to the dying person. Good hospices are places that coordinate care between the mind, the body, the family, and the spirit.

Legal support and impetus for the hospice movement has also been a significant trend in recent years. It started, as is so often the case, with a very human face — that of Karen Ann Quinlan. The year after Connecticut Hospice opened, Karen, at that time only twenty-one years old, was found in a coma at her home in suburban New Jersey. In 1976 her family set legal precedent when they won the right to refuse medical treatment, allowing doctors to remove her from a respirator. But it would take another ten years before Karen died. She remained in a fetal position, wasting from 120 to 68 pounds, subsisting on a feeding tube. Her parents visited her at her nursing home every day.

Eerily, Karen ended up dying — of pneumonia — shortly after the New Jersey State Supreme Court also made it legal for doctors to remove permanently comatose patients from feeding tubes. But the U.S. Supreme Court didn't uphold these decisions until 1990, with the case of Nancy Cruzan. Karen's case was the first indication that people wanted to take back some control over their deaths; many Americans *still* fear a slow death on machinery that makes prolonged life a living hell. In 1991, after thousands of similar cases, the federal government enacted the Patient Self-Determination Act. Now, whenever we enter a medical center, we must be informed of our right to decide our care and be given the opportunity to fill out health-care proxies or living wills. The PSDA has helped people choose hospice, as did a 1983 bill passed by Congress that ensures that hospice is covered through Medicare, Medicaid, and private insurers.

Hospice has brought death home, and with it has come the new understanding of how to bring closure to life. It has helped us appreciate that life is about connections, relationships, family, unconditional love. That is what the photographers in this exhibition saw when they went to visit dying patients. Somehow, we are learning as a nation to talk about death, to hold loved ones' hands, to kiss them, and to say good-bye. Hospice helped us put dying back into the realm of the human.

All of these photographers came to this project with personal experiences of death that shaped their vision and the stories they wanted to tell of dying. But hospice and the people they saw dying significantly moved and changed them, showing them the unexpected, helping them learn that life is about living until the end, that mystical things can happen, and in a way, that all of life is a memory, a dream, of double and triple exposures. As artists, each photographer gave us back a vision of what is now emerging as a modern art of dying.

Sally Mann looked at places — coating them with mystical visions, memories, symbols — the kind of places Audrey envisioned when she was packing her bags for her journey. Mann's photographs — particularly the one of the falling bridge — convey the majesty one feels when confronted with the unknown on the edges of life.

Kathy Vargas's great-aunt, who was a nun, began the first hospice in San Antonio. She took Kathy with her while she visited patients there twenty years ago. The wonder of it stuck with her, but she realized its power only when her own father recently died. Kathy's work seems to superimpose past life, what we make of this life, and an afterlife, one on top of the other, producing both dream and vision.

Jack Radcliffe talks about moments of connection and magic, about finding life at the end of life, and also finding joy. Which is a wonderful play on words, since his hospice guide in York, Pennsylvania, was Joy Ufema, one of the early lights of the American hospice movement. Mystery shapes Joy's own life. She tells the story of working in her garden and finding a letter A — on a child's block in the dirt — a letter that for Joy symbolized AIDS. She took it as a message to start York hospice for AIDS patients. Jack says patients there taught him just the things he needed to learn, since his own mother had just died and his father was in the process of dying.

For Jim Goldberg, it was his father's death that was the focus of his project, so the intimacy of family was primary. Majesty for him was in the details, the things one needs in the intimacy of dying — a urine bottle, an oxygen tank, a hospital bed, a shower — simple things, but they also communicate family caring and love.

Finally, it was Nan Goldin's friend Cookie whose death inspired her participation in this project. Nan was in Berlin, Germany, when Cookie died. She missed her death and heard stories about how powerful it was. Cookie died at Cabrini Hospice, and beside her were her friends and Sister Loretta, helping her through.

In helping people die, Sister Loretta says, it's caring and touch that count, even if it means becoming as exposed and raw as all of us will eventually become in the process of dying ourselves. In the end, love is what matters, a heart connection so real that no one feels afraid to delve into emotional business left unresolved, or fears that they are alone as they die. Yet helping someone like this is a particular kind of challenge, one that modern medicine hasn't well addressed.

In addition to physical pain, there is another kind of suffering in dying — the sadness that comes in realizing you are leaving this earth forever, the sadness of being helpless in the face of decline. This is the pain of permanently leaving home, of leaving family, friends, and children, of saying good-bye to a job, or a beloved dog or cat. It's the pain of no longer being able to go skiing or sailing, or to walk or get on a plane, of not even being able to sit quietly and knit, or lie outside on the grass. Unless this kind of pain is also eased, a person will have difficulty in dying. But when it is well addressed, the sadness can bring something else: a transcendent feeling that can be expanded, changed, enlarged, a certain, very new kind of hope.

One day, Sister Loretta went to sit with a dying patient named Joseph. A young doctor was standing near him. "The doctor didn't know what to do, since he'd done everything he could do medically," she says. "Joseph had signed papers requesting no treatment. I pulled up a chair and began stroking his arm and talking to him gently. The doctor saw a pack of cigarettes on the TV and asked if he could take one. Joseph wouldn't be needing them anymore, so I told him okay, I didn't think he'd mind.

"The doctor went out into the hall, smoking and pacing. He kept looking back in," she says.

"Then he came back and sat there as I sang softly to Joseph and told him, 'Look for your parents. They're going to show you new playgrounds.' Boy, was I nervous. I'd never had a doctor watch me before. But I kept on. All of a sudden, Joseph smiled, tried to sit up, and held out his arms. 'Sister,' he said, 'I see them.' Since I was nervous, I didn't think I heard right, so I asked who. 'My parents,' he said. 'And they're just as beautiful as you said.' Right after that, he died."

Just then, the doctor's beeper went off and he started to run out of the room. Sister Loretta asked if he wanted the cigarettes. He called back that he didn't smoke. She sat with Joseph about ten minutes longer, still stroking him, then she went to find this young doctor. He'd seemed so nervous. "I know you've seen death before," she said.

"Sister," he told her. "I've seen death, but only in emergency situations. It's always been so frenetic and violent. Never so peaceful like that. You know, if people have to die, everyone should be able to die like that."

our engagement
picture

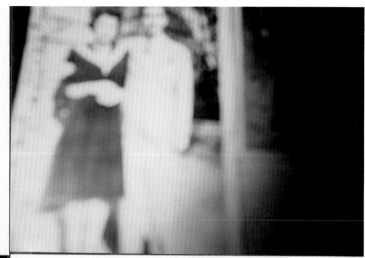

The lemons
on our lemon tree

Dad's favorite room
in the house. I
had his chair moved
out here.

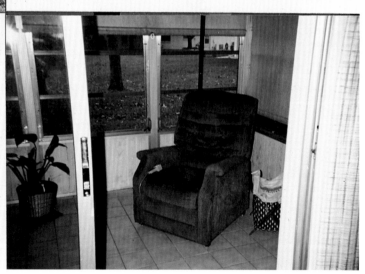

Jim Goldberg
Dad's Favorite Room, 1994

HOSPICE: A Photographic Inquiry
BY JANE LIVINGSTON

The introduction of hospice care into the United States constitutes one of the great quiet revolutions of our time. More and more people in our society are living their last days, or months, in an environment of cooperative interaction with others, expressly so that they might be made comfortable and calm and that they may properly say their good-byes. And yet it is safe to say that the vast majority of Americans have no true idea of what hospice care is all about, especially in the concrete sense of how it affects those whose lives and deaths have been entrusted to it. Since no revolution occurs without education, especially one that touches on something as universal as a society's culture of dying, the challenge facing hospice care at this moment is to communicate what it is all about. Occasionally art serves to educate far more powerfully than any amount of explaining; those of us who entered together into this experiment have often seen it happen.

Hospice: A Photographic Inquiry is a collaborative endeavor between two traditions. One of those, photography, seems merely a ubiquitous fact of life, an ordinary tool for documenting the world, or pieces of it. The other one, that of an unconventional approach to the matter of dying known as hospice, is far less familiar in our current society. Indeed, we may even think of hospice care as a somewhat threatening notion. And yet these two ideas, photography and hospice, have much in common.

As everyday, and ever present, as it may seem, photography itself is still an often-misunderstood tradition, or art — and a fairly recent one. Indeed, photography's history is far shorter than that of hospice. And though nothing can be more ever present than the fact of dying, hospice's way of dealing with this universally experienced event has only recently been widely reengaged. In a sense, photography and hospice share deeply in the qualities of being both quietly revolutionary and misunderstood.

Both hospice and certain photographers work a little subversively, or outside the system. The hospice worker and the photographer each engages in an intimate exchange with other human beings, and both are on double journeys — of self-discovery and of showing new or deeper realities to other people. Both wait for moments of revelation; both need help, from one another and from others, to achieve their ends.

Photography is a tradition just over one hundred fifty years old. Thus, it is a relatively new vehicle both for the examination of the world and for creative expression. It is easy to forget that for the vast part of modern history, humankind functioned without the extraordinarily powerful, yet simple, image-gathering technique whose principle was artfully to expose tiny pieces of "reality" to a surface activated by light and shade, and thereby produce a peculiar trace of something that we, viewing the result, might fully believe existed or happened in space and time. A photograph, it has been said, is not a fiction.

But this claim is true only in a very limited sense. Perhaps a photograph can be said to possess some quality of natural verisimilitude. However, in a more encompassing sense, a photograph is just as subjective an interpretation of "reality" as any of the other visual arts. The author of the photographic image, whether a skilled artist or an amateur — or even a computerized camera programmed by a team of scientists — is the creator of the traces we see on a flat surface. To the extent that the photograph — the image we observe embedded in the silver-coated paper, or printed on the page of the book — does represent some slice of "reality," it is at most a shadowy trace of objects or events altered in profound ways. Through the photographic process, something resembling what we see around us was selected in a viewfinder and exposed. That is the "decisive moment" selected by the artist. After that, the image may be cropped from its original proportions, and certainly it is manipulated in the process of its printing, even if unintentionally.

The result is, by definition, an *interpretation* of things observed, and thus essentially a sort of fiction.

And to the extent that the death of an individual is shared in by others, that event becomes, for all but the deceased, an indelible memory, an occasion with all the detailed reality of life's especially acute experiences. Still, that event, like the aftermath of the photographic exposure, bears only the most fragile connection to the phenomenon that occurred for the individual whose death created the momentous occasion. It is in part this obvious, yet paradoxical, truth that hospice seems to grasp and to use in its own transformative endeavor.

The necessarily interpretive, or metamorphic, nature of the photographic medium, far from reducing its power as an image-making tool, actually heightens its power. And this attribute of photography may be especially potent when the photographer's subject is another person, for then the act of exposing the photograph becomes a collaborative event. Portraiture is one of photography's richest and most enduring traditions; one reason for this has to do with the participatory nature of the photographic portrait, and thus its ability to become at the same time both portrait and self-portrait.

Portrait photography's engagement of the subject of death and dying is by no means a modern phenomenon. One of the medium's earliest professional traditions was the *memento mori*. In nineteenth-century American photography, it was not just the family portrait, but the deathbed portrait, that kept many of the commercial studios in business for several decades. It was not unusual for families during the 1860s, and until after the turn of the century, to commission and display photographs of deceased children, looking (it was hoped) as though in a peaceful sleep. But this aspect of the photographic tradition is clearly a very different thing from the present endeavor.

Hospice, by acknowledging that both the process of dying and the impact of a person's death on the lives of others are matters that affect many individuals, also enables a transformation in people's reality, through collaborative engagement. By seeing the act of dying as a participatory event, and by allowing the process to take its own shape according to the character and choices of the dying person, hospice facilitates a series of metamorphoses. Photography and hospice both can be said to show us realities we didn't know existed — and to remind us that there are as many "truths" as there are individual experiences.

Another sense in which photography is empowered by its own interpretive nature is in its uniquely flexible adaptability to storytelling. Unlike a story or a poem, a photograph needn't refer to anything outside itself to tell its story. Still, many accomplished photographers, whether artists, journalists, or amateurs, possess the gift of narration and can bring a surprising freight of information to one picture. Many of the memorable single images in the history of the medium are dense, and often variously interpretable, with the telling of a story. But photographs can be especially effective in their storytelling capacity when they are conceived and presented in groups or series.

Similarly, anyone who has been exposed to the hospice idea comes to realize that its essence is in allowing the ever-fascinating *stories* of each person's life and death to emerge unforgettably. Our stories are what remain when we are gone.

Then there is the question of the actual text or captions that might or might not accompany photographs and thus complete their meaning. Despite resistance to the idea, some kinds of photographic projects simply require accompanying texts in order to become fully realized. At the very least, certain images fail or succeed by virtue of that simplest of captions, the identification of the subject by name.

Some subjects require much more than a name — many more descriptive or explanatory words — before they become transparent. We experience this every day when we read the newspaper. And yet, at least in the history of photography as an art form, it has not been common to locate subjects through which to marry photographs and verbal stories, so that the two forms of expression become a single, irreplaceable art form. James Agee and Walker Evans's collaborative work, *Let Us Now Praise Famous Men*, that Depression-era classic, is one such example; Eugene Smith's extensively captioned photographic essay *Country Doctor* is another. It may not be coincidental that these artists' subjects are ones dealing with fundamental human predicaments, and with people reaching out to each other to illuminate or assuage them.

In the period of photography's awakening as a recognized art form — roughly the 1960s and 1970s — exhibitions rarely included "photo stories" or even individual images with lengthy texts. It was not (nor is it today) unusual for art photographs to be untitled. This modernist fashionability of the monolithic and self-referential object began in the 1980s to be replaced with a postmodernist emphasis on image-and-text as interdependent. In the wake of a decade-long period of postmodernist experiments combining pictures and language (a use of words that tended to be cryptic and only marginally narrative), some photographers lately are reengaging a more old-fashioned use of text in relation to images.

Recent customs surrounding death and dying in the United States have evolved through a similar process, from being treated silently to being (largely through the presence of hospice) more actively accepted and, in a sense, named. During an era of rapid and dramatic changes in medical technology, the last half-century or so when more patients returned from hospitals and medical centers cured, or improved, than dying, the treatment of death itself became, in a sense, disassociated from its own story. The story was the cure or healing of the body, not the ending of the life. For many years in our society, easy conversation, or storytelling, about most people's deaths simply disappeared. The freeing narrative creativity in relation to death associated with several earlier immigrant cultures — such as those elaborate stories told to each other by slaves or among Irish-Americans — seemed to go underground. Deathbed stories were buried along with the body of the deceased. Hospice rejects this burying of the unique story of each person's death. Aside from its many other contributions, this reborn tradition has already helped to restore language and storytelling to the tradition of death and dying.

*I*t is plain to anyone contemplating this commissioned exhibition called *Hospice: A Photographic Inquiry* that it represents a high-risk experiment. The idea offered the opportunity for collaboration between two sympathetic traditions. And yet there were no guarantees that it would succeed as an exhibition and book. To have a chance at success, the experiment required the participation of especially gifted and experienced artists, and an extraordinary amount of cooperation on the part of many hospice organizations. In formulating this exhibition, we — Dena Andre, Philip Brookman, Frances Fralin, and I — were acutely aware that not every photographer would be willing to take on the kind of assignment we were proposing. Besides being equipped to work for a sustained period with individuals in situations that by definition presented unpredictable circumstances and events, each of the five artists would, we felt, need to be especially adept at communicating the stories implicit in the images they were capturing. We were also determined that the five photographers would each use an entirely different approach from the others.

As events transpired, we were soon able to agree on the five individuals we hoped would accept our invitation to this challenge. Miraculously, each of our candidates eventually agreed. The separate approaches taken by these five artists have become something like a demonstration of what it is possible to do in the photographic essay. Ranging from the familiar documentary approach to highly metaphoric imagery, these few bodies of work hint at the enormous range of possibility in the use of the camera, by itself or with accompanying language, to transform intense experience into artistic expression.

*P*hotographic images and words don't easily combine to form coherent works of art. One of the most inventive approaches to the problem of language/image synthesis is that of Jim Goldberg in his riveting series of works, *Rich and Poor,* made during the late 1970s and 1980s. In them, the photographer presented his own black-and-white photographs of individuals — young and old, in contrasting economic circumstances, in dramatically varying environments — superimposed with their own handwritten comments about these pictures.

It is a stunning device, carried off with apparent simplicity and naturalness. With a single stroke, Goldberg has created images that are literally both portraits and self-portraits, but that also introduce a new element, or layer, of meaning — namely, the exteriorized contrast between our own ("objective") view of the person depicted (or, perhaps more accurately, Jim Goldberg's view) and the photographic subject's own view of that depiction.

Goldberg moved on from this extended experiment to several photographic ideas that are less literally documentary, notably an extended work, titled *Raised by Wolves,* about runaway children in California living (and dying) together in reconstructed "families" in various streets and parks and abandoned buildings. In this highly experimental effort, the artist moved into ever more intricate psychological terrain, elaborating on his earlier technique of allowing photographed subjects to provide their own stories and finding ways to allow his subjects to interact with him and each other in the structuring of his work.

One of Goldberg's trademarks is the seemingly raw, or improvisational, style of his imagery. He has found ways to allow his images to remain in a strikingly informal state, usually juxtaposed with other images and with words whose presentation is equally informal — and to use these qualities of a sort of calculated randomness, or casualness, to carry much of the aesthetic weight of his presentations. It is as though his photographs and their sometimes quite elaborate captions have grown organically out of a cumulative process, like the making of a family album or a personal journal.

During the period when Goldberg was working on *Raised by Wolves,* his own father was terminally ill with cancer. When it became clear that his disease would inevitably progress, Herbert Goldberg and his family decided that, as much as possible, he would remain at home, and they turned to the Suncoast Hospice organization in their Florida community. Jim Goldberg, living and working in San Francisco, visited his father as often as he could and recorded what transpired as this proud and vivid man gradually relinquished his hold on life. The son's documenting of his father's illness and death would result in the memorable body of work we see here, becoming an eloquent photographic meditation on the subject of the father/son bond, and on its physical ending.

It is crucial to the story of Herbert Goldberg's dying that it took place at home. Everything about this drama — the images of the man himself and the particulars of his environment, unmistakably that of an ill person determined to preserve the familiar; the people around him, sharing his home or providing company and care; the memoirs and letters of the story's main characters, providing a glimpse into their sometimes ambivalent relationships; and the son's recollection of his father's very last moments — seems intimate, specific to the last detail, and remarkably universal.

It is clear when we explore these words and images that something besides the dying man and his family is present in this environment, some sustaining force that is making it possible for this drama to be unfolding in a domestic milieu. That presence is, of course, hospice. The interaction of many individuals — family members and friends, hospice staff and volunteers — becomes as much a subject of the photographer's work as the passing away of its central character.

The photographer and his family have provided the skill and the generosity to allow Herbert Goldberg's story to become universal; the institution of hospice has created the conditions for this artistic transformation. The lessons of hospice have helped make it possible for the dying man and his family to acknowledge and explore the event confronting them — and have given us, the viewers of the completed work, the permission and the courage to participate in the death of a man we never knew and to glimpse his son's loss.

Nan Goldin made her entry onto the photographic scene in 1985 with a remarkable body of work she called *The Ballad of Sexual Dependency*. This extended photographic essay, which combined fact and fiction, personal narrative and imaginary stories, was achieved over a period of years and is dedicated to the artist's sister, Barbara, who committed suicide at the age of eighteen. The original work was shown as a slide presentation at the Whitney Museum, and released as a book the next year. The *Ballad* continues to exist in a constantly changing form, presented as projected slides and as various exhibitions of prints. Goldin managed, with this innovative body of work, to forge a new range of possibilities for the still camera by virtue of her unflinching eye and her habit of inserting herself — both emotionally and physically — into the scenario. The fluidity of incident and the strong atmosphere of autobiography that characterizes the extended *Ballad* seem to have established a kind of departure point for her work ever since. Goldin has continued to work with the same passionate engagement of subjects close to her own life, including a long photographic essay dealing with three good friends' experience living with and dying from AIDS.

Nan Goldin's mastery of color in photography as an emotionally defining pictorial element — combined with her essentially documentary, unstaged stylistic approach — gives to her work an emotional intensity and truthfulness that are peculiarly her own. She has a rare capacity to make her chromatic palette do different things at the same time, seeming, for example, at once lush and bleak. Beyond these physical qualities lies a more subtle one. The artist's willingness to project herself, her own desires and fears, into her images lends to her photographs, especially when viewed cumulatively, an aura of immediacy and truth that are rare in any artistic medium.

Until recently, Goldin's work has been undertaken in the spirit of an enormously candid and searching diary. Her subjects have been the people and events in her own life. Virtually for the first time, Goldin worked with people unknown to her beforehand for this project. Making occasional, highly focused visits to the homes of patients cared for by Cabrini Hospice in Manhattan, she became acquainted with and photographed a wide range of subjects over the period of a year and a half. The individuals vary in age and circumstance, ranging from thirty-five-year-old Joseph, dying of AIDS, to forty-year-old Amalia, terminally ill with cancer. Given the brevity of the photographer's periods of contact with these people, their subjects' air of absolute frankness, of fragile selves being revealed without hesitation, becomes something of a mystery. The subjects of these pictures seem somehow to have been asked, and to have deliberately agreed, to give of themselves at a profound level. It is as if they are engaged in creative acts, showing their most definitive and uncensored self to someone whom they recognize and trust.

Typical of the manner in which she has become accustomed to approaching her stories, the photographer has gravitated to her subjects' physical environments and to the relationships in each one's life, to fashion a view of the whole person. Many images in each cumulative portrait depict a bedside tabletop or objects hung on a wall or a visiting child. The absence of the protagonist in certain images serves to flesh out the larger picture. With a few deft strokes, Nan Goldin tells a series of strangely resonant tales, bringing into keen focus a number of individuals whose present consciousness is clearly being experienced with a heightened sensibility. The awareness of time's preciousness, especially in scenes where her subjects are responding to the presence of others, is conveyed with an acute immediacy.

Sally Mann's entire artistic impulse has sometimes seemed a sort of tug-of-war between her natural gifts as a writer and her better-known photographic achievement. Although Mann's many exhibitions and several books have primarily centered on visual images, virtually everything she has done has been accompanied by a carefully crafted textual record, whether through notes to herself or correspondence with others. In identifying Mann as an artist who might rise to the occasion presented by this commissioned project, it was with the hope that she would combine her literary abilities with her photographic expertise.

Like Nan Goldin, Sally Mann has tended to center her photographic work on people close to her in her everyday life. In Mann's case, family members and friends in her native town of Lexington, Virginia, where she still lives, have inspired much of her best work. Perhaps her most intimate photographic engagement with another human being came about with the death of her father in 1988. Suffering from brain cancer, he elected, with the help of the local hospice, to remain at home. His daughter recorded the event of his death by depicting its immediate aftermath.

From her 1988 book, *At Twelve: Portraits of Young Women*, to the many extraordinary images of her own children, resulting in the book *Immediate Family* in 1992, Mann's lyrical yet psychologically penetrating, often dreamlike, photographs have added a distinctive voice to the literature of recent photography. A unique approach combining a mythic, and sometimes downright romantic, undertone with a clear-eyed investigative spirit gives to Mann's photographs, particularly those presented in series, the character of poignant reports on how it is to exist in another person's skin.

For Mann, the decision to embark on a journey into the world of the dying, though not easy to make, was finally arrived at because in the course of her father's last illness, she had made a new friend in Joan Robins. Robins is a professional nurse at the Rockbridge Area Hospice. Rockbridge hospice is an organization dedicated solely to providing at-home, or other outpatient, care and support. At a time when Mann was ready to make a change in her work, turning away from her most intimate circle of subjects to focus on a more anonymous universe, her relationship to Joan Robins and the proposed commission for this project seemed finally to suggest a possible way to work that would be different from anything attempted before.

Of all the artists in this group, Mann has most taken it upon herself to find out what it is that

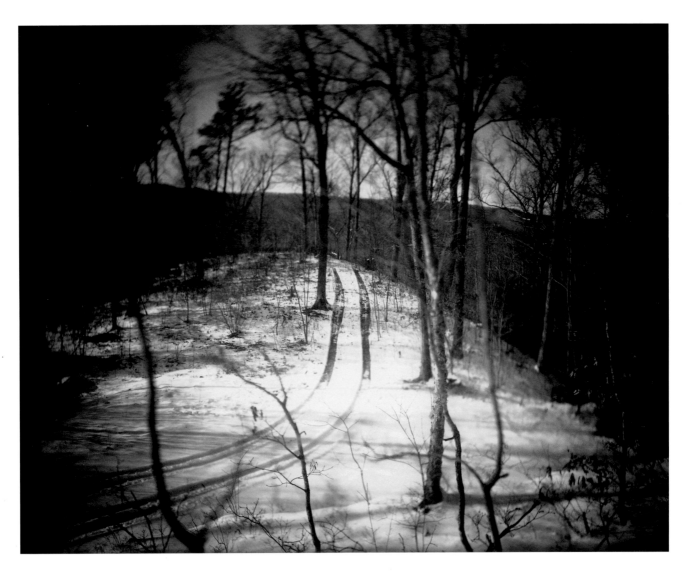

Sally Mann
Untitled, 1994 from
Vinculum: What Matters

One patient wanted only to
revisit the place where,
with bow and arrow,
he'd killed his first deer.

the ultimate teachers of the hospice movement — those facing the ends of their lives on earth — might see or feel. Meeting each of her subjects, Mann absorbs what she can of their desires and memories. Through a series of imaginative acts taking as a starting point a view from a window, or a recollected favorite place, she then uses her camera to reconstruct something telling about the lives of the people to whom she has been introduced by Joan. In the course of her investigations, many individuals are swept into the web of her observations, and the great questions about the brevity of everyone's time in this life — and everyone's experience of the loss of others — become the subject of the artist's inquiry. The photographs here become more like talismans than portraits or descriptive documents. They represent a departure for this artist. Even without the words that elucidate their imagery, we, their viewers, are never in doubt about what theme underlies their conception. Rather than the quick ripeness that characterizes so much of Mann's other work, these meditative images evince a stillness that can only signal the presence of death.

Of all the photographers in the present company, the one whose efforts for this book and exhibition have persisted the longest is Jack Radcliffe. His commitment has been different from the rest in both its duration and its singlemindedness. For a period of some three years, Radcliffe has made frequent and regular visits to one small hospice, York House in York, Pennsylvania, and has worked closely with its founder and chief administrator, Joy Ufema. The relationship between Radcliffe and Ufema, and their mutual discoveries in the task of interacting with a series of patients, is at the core of the work Radcliffe has forged through his association with our project. The two of them have taught the rest of us a great deal about the phenomenon of hospice.

Jack Radcliffe is in one sense the most traditional of our five photographers in his use of photography. For as many years as he has been working and teaching — since 1978 — he has confined his work to black-and-white imagery, using a Hasselblad camera and limiting himself to a rigorously classical and highly disciplined vocabulary in composing and printing his pictures. Radcliffe has centered his work on the environment in which he has lived for most of his life, Baltimore, Maryland, and its surrounding rural or small-town areas. But he has gone into hidden places, finding entrance to the homes and cultures of such marginal groups as Ku Klux Klan cadres or others of the slightly less dispossessed lower middle classes. His work has always been characterized by a distinctive sense of intimacy with his subjects and a remarkable glimpsing of private, even secret, scenes or startlingly exposed psychological states not often caught by the camera.

The hallmark of Radcliffe's work, compared with others who use a similarly conservative technical approach and who concentrate primarily on candid, documentary photography, is the formidable compassion and insight he brings to everything he does. Rarely does one find that quality of the cold, or "objective," observation of ordinary people in everyday life that is so often associated with the kind of photography he does. Occasionally Radcliffe transcends even the rarefied level of empathy he brings to virtually all of his work, seeming to find a path inside his subjects; in some of his photographs, one imagines that the author is looking out of the image at himself.

Like other photographers in this project, Radcliffe was led to an interest in the hospice movement through personal experience. In 1991 his mother died of cancer, and after that, as his father's health declined, he found himself having to prepare for that loss as well. The necessity of forming relationships with patients at York House Hospice that would enable him to achieve the kind of potent and self-revelatory images he wanted to make in some way helped him, he says, to understand and to accept his own more fundamental losses. However, his work with AIDS patients has been far from an easy undertaking. Radcliffe often established bonds with people he sometimes knew for only a few days, though often much longer. That caused him to suffer when they died. Most of his subjects were too young to be facing death. He learned their stories and met their children, parents, and friends, and often came to understand all too well the burden of their loss.

Radcliffe's images made at York House Hospice are probably some of the most difficult to view. Even when his pictures center on the touching connection between two individuals preparing to be separated, as in those showing Larry and Frank, or Rogen and Dave together, they pierce to the raw heart of terrible illness. More than any of the other images in this project, Radcliffe's communicate the overwhelming effort demanded of the patient by the call to live, to respond to others, when one is sick unto death.

All of the individuals photographed by Jack Radcliffe were suffering with AIDS; most of them came to York House from humble circumstances; many had led lives of extraordinary insecurity and deprivation. One of the many amazing attributes of Radcliffe's perception of these people, given the difficulties of their lives past and present, is the sheer vividness of their presence, the sharp individuality and fierce humanity elicited by the camera. Even without knowing the stories of the wonderful child Boo Boo, or the unforgettably proud and quick-witted Sheila, we feel in these mute pictures an almost eerie sense of the life-pulse, and the struggle of those captured in them.

Although Jack Radcliffe's pictures have a look of inevitability, as though they had composed themselves, in fact they are authoritatively crafted. Part of his technique relies on an insistent monumentality of composition, combined with a strong linear drive. His lens reaches right up into the gesture. Mass works in counterpoint with contour. For instance, in each image of the handsome, long-limbed Sheila, the angles of her body and the objects around her, the strong diagonals and curves of each outline in the picture, build a structure emphasizing the key visual element of her and of the picture — her huge, expressive eyes. As we analyze each image, we discover that each employs this same principle of locating some very particular feature — whether a way of posturing the arms or body, or a distinctive droop of the jaw — and intuitively presents that feature through artfully empathic, rather than psychologically confrontational, means.

Here again, as in the work of Jim Goldberg, the pictures reflect a reality outside their boundaries. It is as though the presence of the hospice workers behind the scenes, the unceasing support of their patients' efforts to be aware and to be comfortable, enters the pictorial ambience despite the single-minded concentration on the physical particularities of the people being photographed.

*T*he work of Kathy Vargas has emerged from different traditions than those informing the other four artists in *Hospice: A Photographic Inquiry*. Vargas, who is of Mexican-American descent, has for many years lived and worked in San Antonio, Texas. Her own heritage, and that of her cultural environment, has as its natural vocabulary a way of dealing with death and remembrance that comes out of an ancient set of rituals. The long Hispanic/Catholic protocol of last rites, and the subsequent ceremonial leave-taking of the dead, have been merged throughout the postconquest era with various Mexican-Indian rituals and attitudes. These Hispano-indigenous traditions have, in turn, been transformed in the process of their transposition into Mexican-American cultures.

There may be no more richly decorous traditions for commemorating the dead than those of certain Mexican-American communities in the Southwest U.S. Latin America's *Dia de los Muertos* — Day of the Dead — is observed by many on this side of the border. It is a celebration with an opulent visual legacy: sugar skulls, wooden skeletons, lacy paper banners, flowers (especially roses and marigolds), and profusions of candles burnt for those not forgotten. And the custom of making home altars — sometimes called *nichos* or *ofrendas* — to commemorate various saints, the Holy Virgin, or deceased members of one's own family, has been continued in many forms by Mexican-Americans. Indeed, the custom of building accretive shrines incorporating humbly allegorical objects and photographs has created the basis for a popular art form that has found its way into the mainstream of American contemporary culture.

To locate and assemble a few strong reminders of a life relinquished, and thus ritualize its passing, is to some extent to ease the survivors' sense of isolation in the face of loss. But this is not to say that to share or entrust one's memories to another is any less delicate a matter in a highly communal tradition like that of Mexico than it is to give our memories to others within cultures used to a more secretive and individualistic response to death.

Kathy Vargas's direct experience with the notion of *recuerdamente* (remembrance) has helped her to understand the difficulties and nuances involved in the various human transactions implicit in the hospice experience. She says that, like the other artists working on this project, her own losses, especially those of her father, her grandmother, and several friends who died of AIDS, helped to prepare her to reach outward to a greater number of people dealing with death and dying. Her relationship to hospices in Austin and San Antonio — especially to Dr. Marian Primomo, who founded the hospice movement in San Antonio — brought her close to the process of death in a way nothing else could. "Hospice is all about relieving pain," she says. "But there's one other thing that's just as important. It gives you a way to say good-bye."

Vargas set out systematically to create shrines in the form of three collaged images disposed as triptychs — or in three cases, a five-part work — to each of the hospice subjects she encountered. Each carefully assembled work was completed after the death of the person being memorialized. This involved dealing not only with the dying patients and hospice staff but, even more important, with the families who had to say good-bye and to remember. Her approach to each situation was different, simply because each family had its own memories and grief. Her task was to come to such a level of trust that her judgment in making the shrine to each deceased person would be accepted by the family members whose words, images, and mementos she used. Only through the process of arriving at an unconditional, mutual confidence would the finished work succeed.

The poetic multipart works created by Vargas separate themselves from the other photographic work in this project in several respects. First, they are made within a distinct and intricate visual tradition, relying on symbols and metaphors more than on ordinary portraiture or documentation. Second, they take their point of departure at a later moment in the hospice-supported process than the rest: they are created in the aftermath of separation. They are objects that connect the living to the actually remembered dead and also bring those of us, for whom the individuals being celebrated are anonymous, into the circle of their remembrance. "What is a photograph," asks Vargas, "if it is not a memory? My feelings about death have always been calm. But this experience has made me hope that my own death comes with some warning. I'd like time to say good-bye to people and to think about what will be remembered."

JIM GOLDBERG

Philip Brookman: Describe your project.

Jim Goldberg: At the same time my family was deciding that my parents needed hospice care, I was offered a commission to create new work about hospice. I had great reservations about doing this, and I felt personally conflicted; however, I decided I should document the process of my father's death. I chronicled it in many different ways. I used photographs, video, and my diary. It all fit together so perfectly because I was able to be with my parents during my father's final days and experience hospice firsthand. As an artist, it made no sense for me to look at somebody else's death when my father's life and death were events I had to come to terms with.

PB: What did you want to accomplish when you started?

JG: I wanted to create a diary of our experience and somehow explore the universal aspects of my father's story. But I didn't know if I could or should make him into a universal father. I didn't know if I could reconcile who he was and who he wasn't. In the end, that didn't matter. I grew to understand him better. It was an honor for me to be there for him. His grace, courage, and actions made him into a wonderful role model.

PB: Did this project help you to examine your own role as a father?

JG: Yes. Around the time that we found out my father was dying, my daughter Ruby was born. There is something about the dying process that's like a birth. I was between two generations, watching and helping during my father's struggle to die, while Ruby was learning to live and walk. I watched, listened to, and learned from Dad, Ruby, my family, and hospice.

PB: Has your understanding of hospice changed through this project?

JG: Of course. Most of my knowledge about hospice came through the experience of working collaboratively with my family and hospice staff. Hospice was our safety net. They were the given, the trust. Hospice became an integral part of our lives. It was the antithesis of how the medical profession works.

PB: Has your understanding of photography changed?

JG: I had to wonder if the camera would distance me from my father. There's no doubt that when you put something physically between yourself and what's happening, it will shield you. My work allowed me to be there. It acted as a focusing mechanism, a discipline that I could use to help me see and feel clearly. In effect, photography intensified the experience.

PB: Is it possible to photograph or to record the passing of life?

JG: Who knows? I could feel something when my father died, but I couldn't see it. I knew there was nothing I could do to show that moment, other than to literally say, "This is it." I photographed the time on my watch the instant my dad died. That picture is so succinct. Through it, I can experience that moment again. I can remember I was there. And perhaps others can experience it too. The bottom line is that it's important to be there for our families, whether it's with a camera or without one.

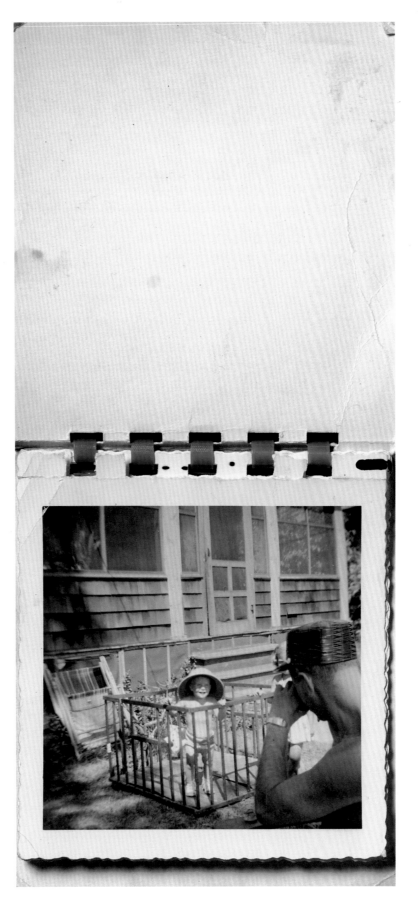

Woodmont, Connecticut
ca. 1955

June, 1989

Dear Jim;

     I have decided to send you a letter containing things
I rememember about you and your young years. I remeber how
excited we were to have a beautiful tow-haired boy who was
spoiled by his brother & sister. How much fun we all had
trying to keep up with a veratible dynamo as you grew up.
How we had to rush you to the emergency room the night y u
ingested a bottle of baby aspirin and had to have your
stomach pumped and how you screamed. How I tried to get you
interested in playing basketball all to no avail and how you
fought against it.
     H w you at one of our anniversary parties insisted
that you must have lobster.
     How, after having your tonsils removed you insisted on
going on a trip with your buddies and how you had to return
in the middle of the night because you were hemmoraging.
     How you ran away to Rabbi Silver's house in Hartford
and how we had to beg you to come home.
     How you argued with me one night; how you ran out of
the house and I tried to catch you and you wound up in New
York at Glenn's.
     How you played hookey from school .
     How you got arrested for stealing a sign off a pole in
front of a policemans house and how we had to go to court
to get the charge squashed.
     How upset you were when I had a nervous breakdown and
wound up in the hospital.
     How angry you were because we thought you were too young
to attend my mothers funeral
     Most of all, I remember one night walking with you and
your telling me all about the stars and planets when I
 realized that were indeed very bright and knowledgable
even though you fought reading.
You have made our life very interesting; we are very proud
 of all that you have accomplished and we love you very dearly.

                                   Your loving father

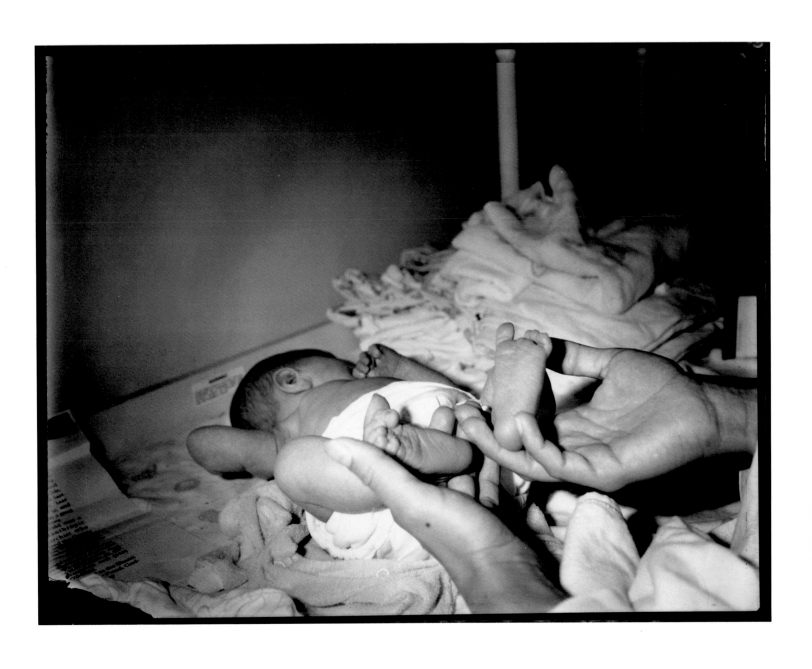

December 12, 1992,
San Francisco, California

April 12, 1993

I am lying on the bed playing with Ruby Sophia, and there is this moment when we look into each other's eyes and she smiles at me and I swoon with memories of myself as a child looking into my father's eyes, doing the same thing. Then the phone rings and it's him, in his bed, weak-voiced. My daddy is dying.

April 17

This is Ruby's first plane flight. At the airport we find my mom at the bottom of the escalator, waiting impatiently for us to discover her more wrinkled face. "It's not so easy taking care of your father anymore," she says. I think she was trying to make a joke.

My father is outside in the front passenger seat of their big pale yellow car. We hug and I can hardly feel his grip on me. I smell his piss bottle hidden in a plastic bag somewhere below his legs. Dad doesn't look sick. His face is full, not wrinkled like Mom's. She sits in the back seat with Susan and tries to play with Ruby. Dad isn't saying much. I drive and try to make conversation and jokes. They become empty one-liners. There is silence, except for Ruby-girl, who is too young to know better.

The Disease

In 1943, during his physical for the draft, my father was diagnosed with a rare degenerative muscle disease. The doctors told him that the syringomyelia would cripple and kill him within a few years. Since then, Dad has lived in defiance of his worsening disability. He was never willing to let others know about his handicap. He used to tell me people thought he was a drunk because of the funny way he walked. In 1984 my father was diagnosed with colon cancer. Six years later, the cancer had spread to his lungs.

For as long as I could remember, Aunt Freda always said, "It's a miracle that Herbie has weathered such an awful storm. I mean look at the man. You would never know he was so sick." She usually said this loudly, behind my father's back.

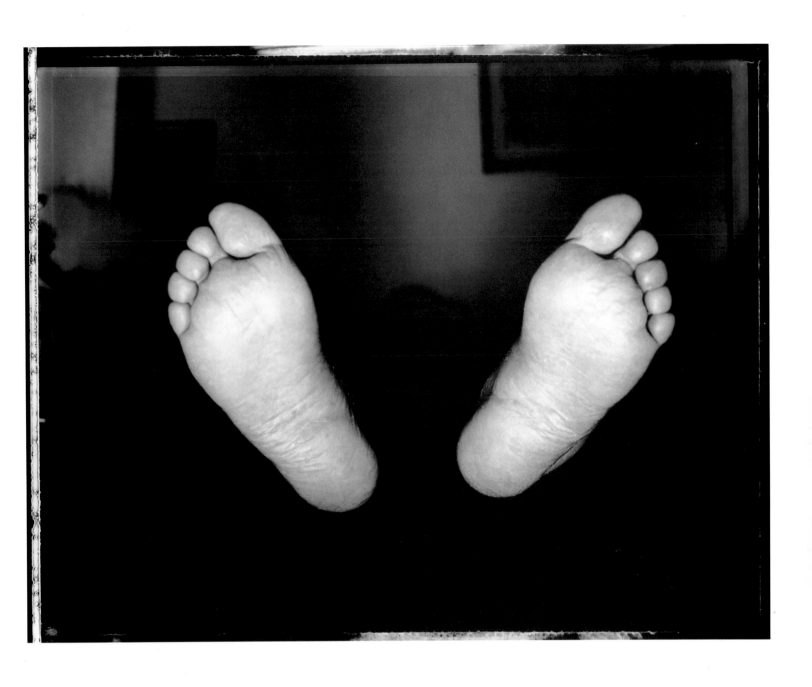

December 19, 1992,
Palm Harbor, Florida

pages 30–31, *Piss Bottle*, 1992–93

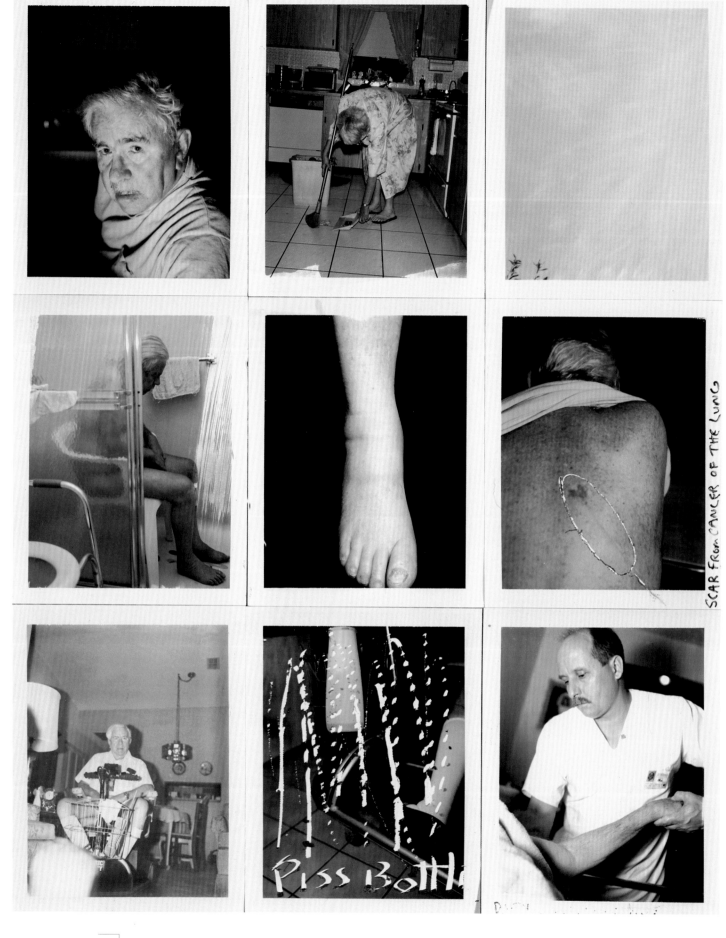

SCAR FROM CANCER OF THE LUNG

Piss Bottle

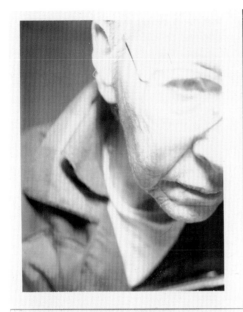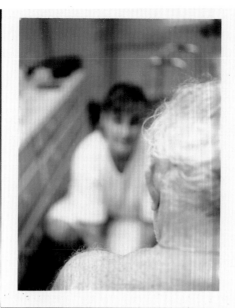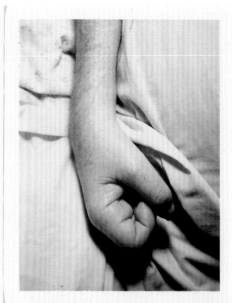
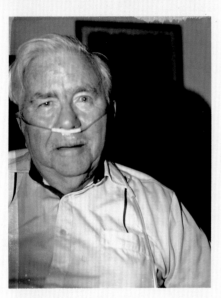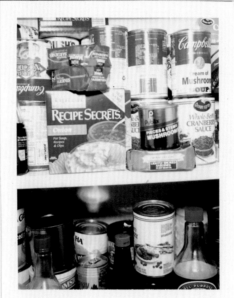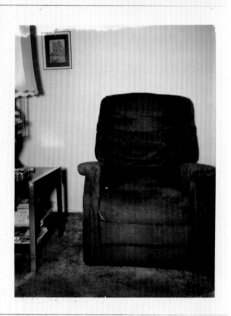
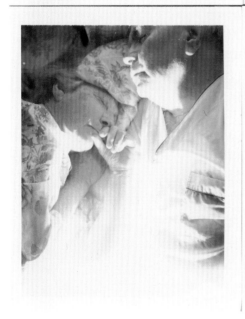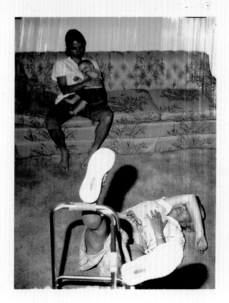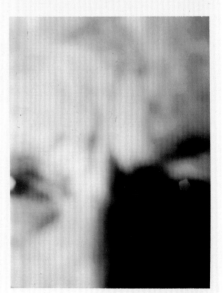

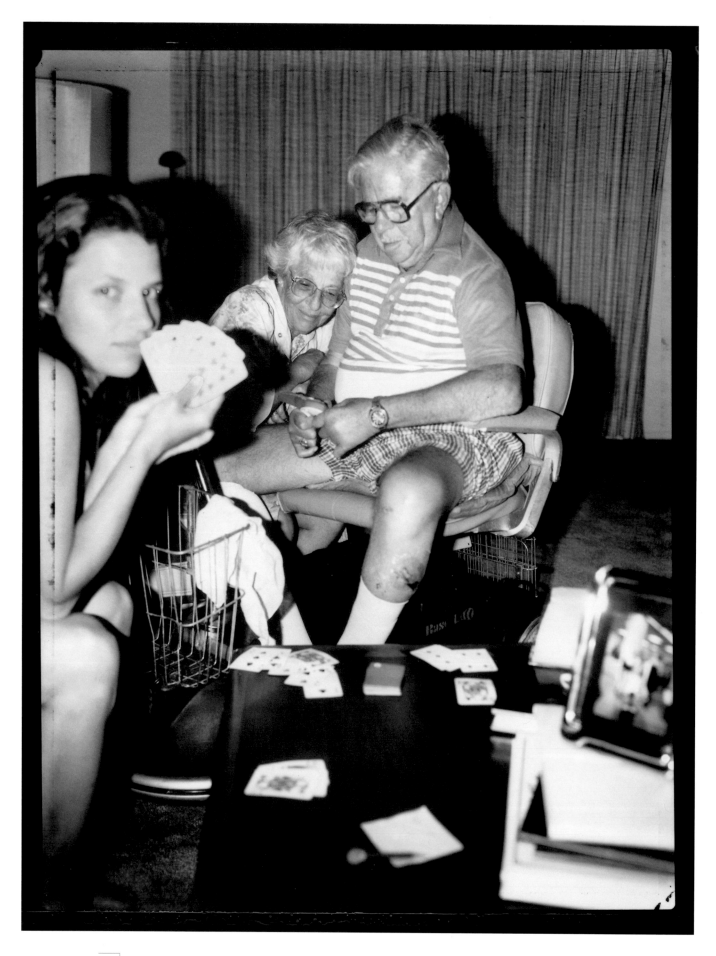

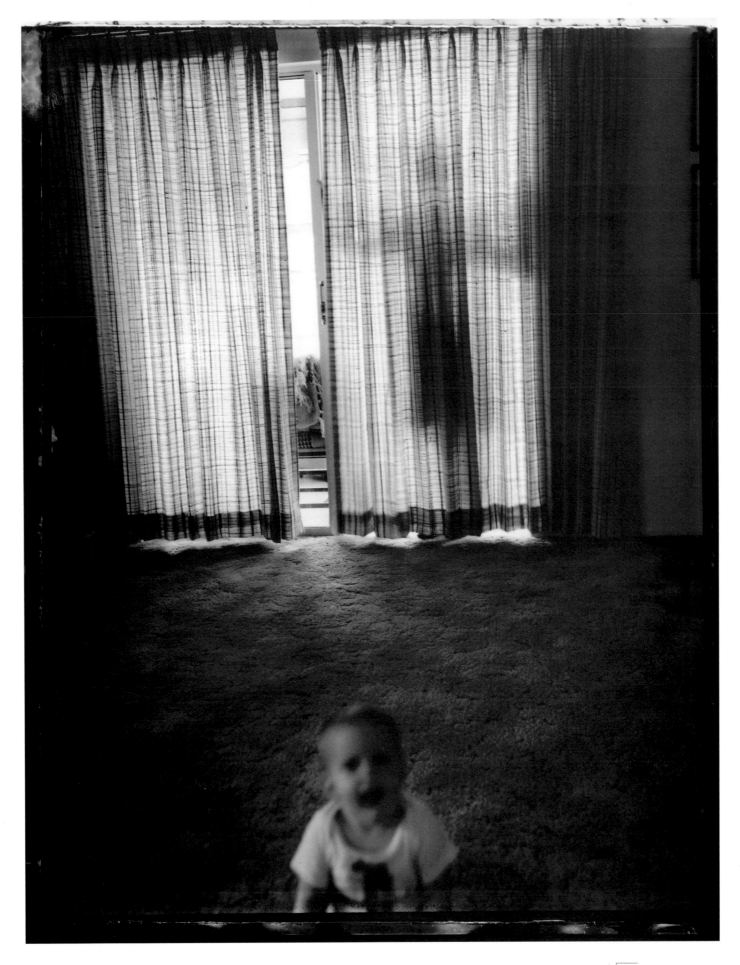

August 17 — Early Morning

Dad has trouble getting back onto his motorized cart. He becomes defeated and self-pitying. Fran, the hospice aide, puts her arms around him and hugs him hard, reminding him in the most unsappy way that hospice is "about living to the fullest and comfortably to the end." My father smiles at her and replies, "Bullshit." She gently rubs lotion on his arms and legs and dresses him. All the while, he gives her driving directions and advice on love and VCR programming.

After Fran leaves, Dad drives his cart to the kitchen table to eat his breakfast, read the paper, and do the crossword puzzle. Dad loves bacon. Mom microwaves it months before it will be served, then freezes it. She microwaves the bacon again to defrost it, then fries it a bit. Sometimes this process happens twice over before it reaches the table. She says she does this "to make sure it's cooked just right, just like your father likes it." Because today is their fifty-second wedding anniversary, Mom has made a mound of bacon. She says, teasingly, "All for my sweetheart, so don't touch any, Jimmy. Okay?"

Dad asks if I want to photograph him with his oxygen, as if the camera is an excuse to play a game of make-believe between father and son. He is obviously out of breath.

The oxygen is kicking in, and his voice becomes stronger. He becomes aware of the camera and vainly attempts to pull his stomach muscles in. But he has no muscles left. Dad says, "You know, Jim, I used to be even skinnier than you when I was a singer. Yes sir, I was a real looker. Do you know what I really want to do now? I want to smoke a cigarette and sing in a karaoke bar."

My father's dreams of a singing career were halted by several things: his marriage, the syringomyelia, his subsequent 4-F draft status, the war, and his decision to take over the family candy business. I first discovered he could lie when I found out that he actually wasn't a secretary on a submarine with Ernest Borgnine.

I ask Dad what he thinks of hospice. "They are very nice people, but it's not me who needs them. It's your mother," he says.

That Afternoon — It's Hot

In the kitchen, Mom defrosts some sandwich meat for lunch. She mumbles, "Your father keeps saying, 'I'm dying. I'm dying.'" She looks down and confesses, "He won't allow me to talk to anybody about his 'condition.' No one knows about hospice. I have to take care of him twenty-four hours a day, and who is going to take care of me if I get sick? I have no one to complain to except hospice. If it weren't for them, I wouldn't have any relief. I don't know if I can take much more, Jimmy. I often think that I want your father to die peacefully — but soon! I know it's normal to feel this way, but still I feel like an awful person having these thoughts."

TV

At night we watch TV. We're all thirsty. I make cold drinks. The freezer compartment is so jammed that it's possible something will fall out and crush my toe. It smells like a luncheonette, but I'm hot, so I forget that the ice in my drink will taste like onions.

page 32, *A Good Moment*, 1992

page 33, *Ruby and Mom*, 1993

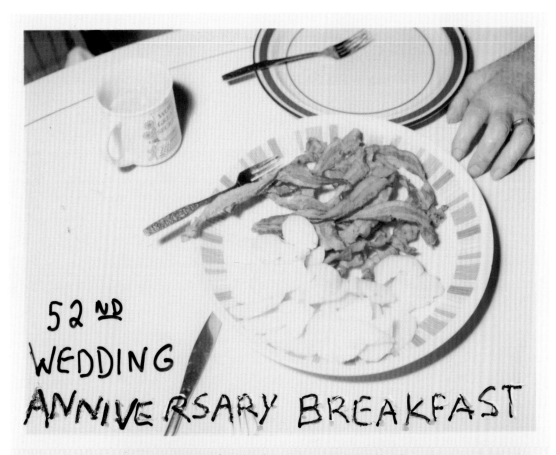

52 ND
WEDDING
ANNIVERSARY BREAKFAST

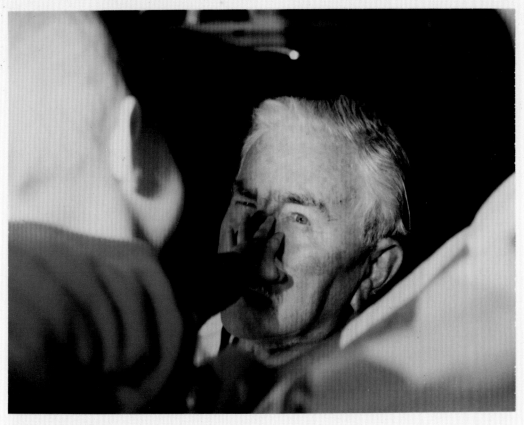

August 17, 1993

pages 36–37
Fran and Herb, 1993

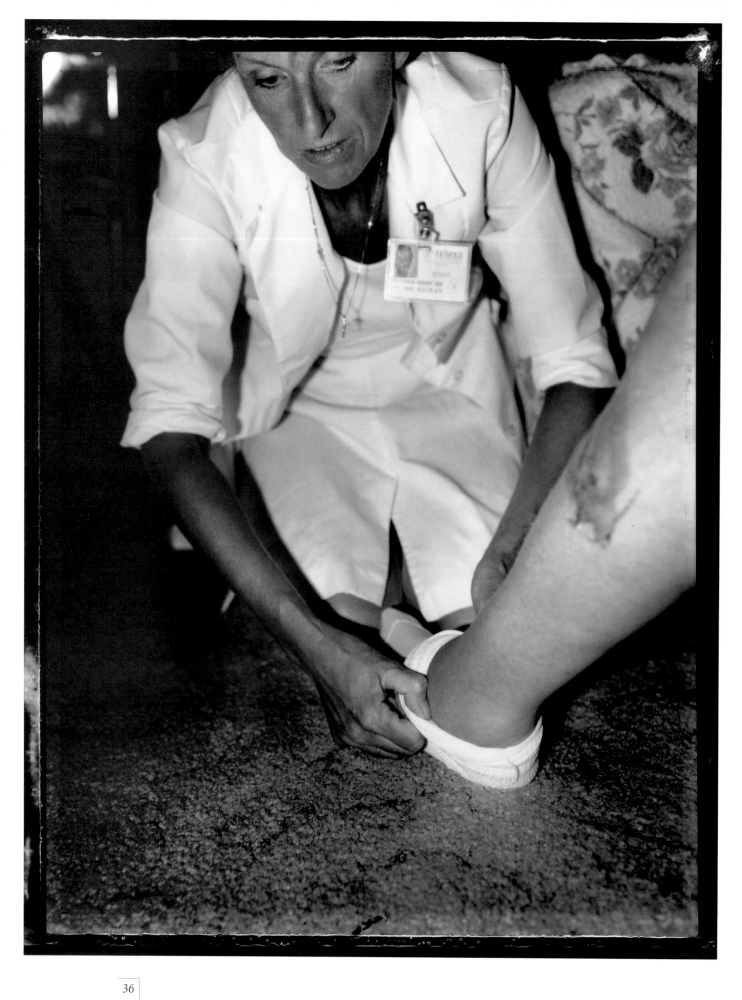

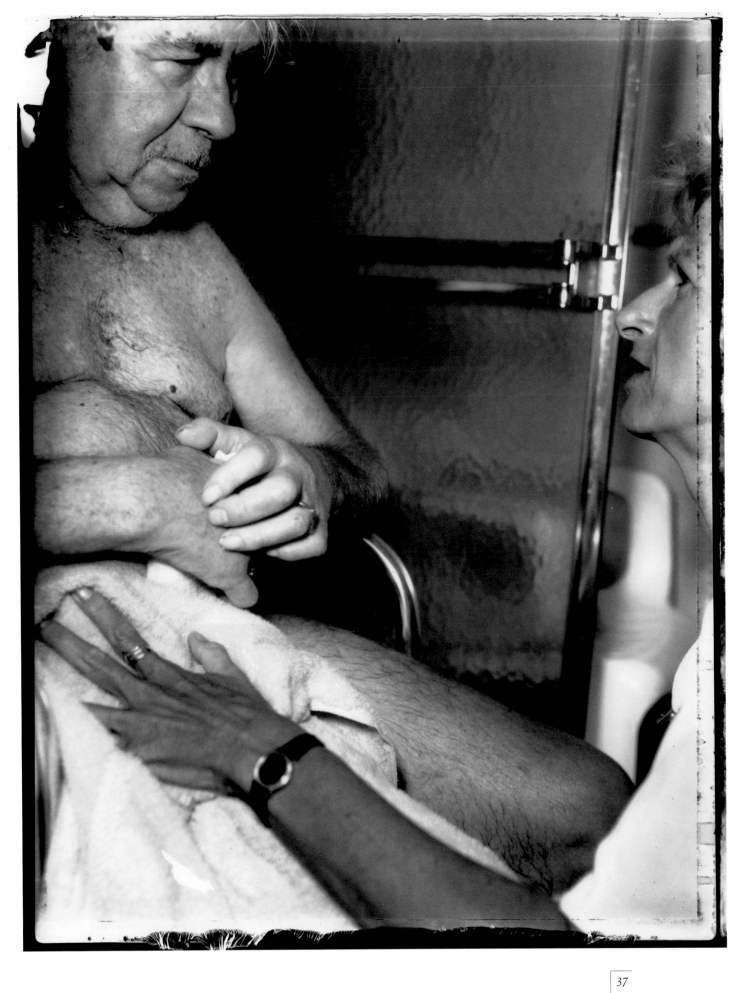

Dr. Ellis + ~~Dr~~ ordered thru Hospice
an evaluation Therapist for Dad. —
Carol called

The man called last night. He's
coming this afternoon — The Therapist
came, nice gentleman but couldn't
help Dad. He suggested exercise but
Dad said exercise tires him out —
Too bad, but we'll work on Therapy
idea when Carol comes next week —
Everyone from Hospice try to help us —
This afternoon they came (without
our calling) to check the oxygen
machine. Making sure it's working
properly — They left us bottles and
tube replacements — I don't know who
called Carol, or Hospice office to
have the machine checked. They
are something.!!

Untitled Video Stills, 1992–93

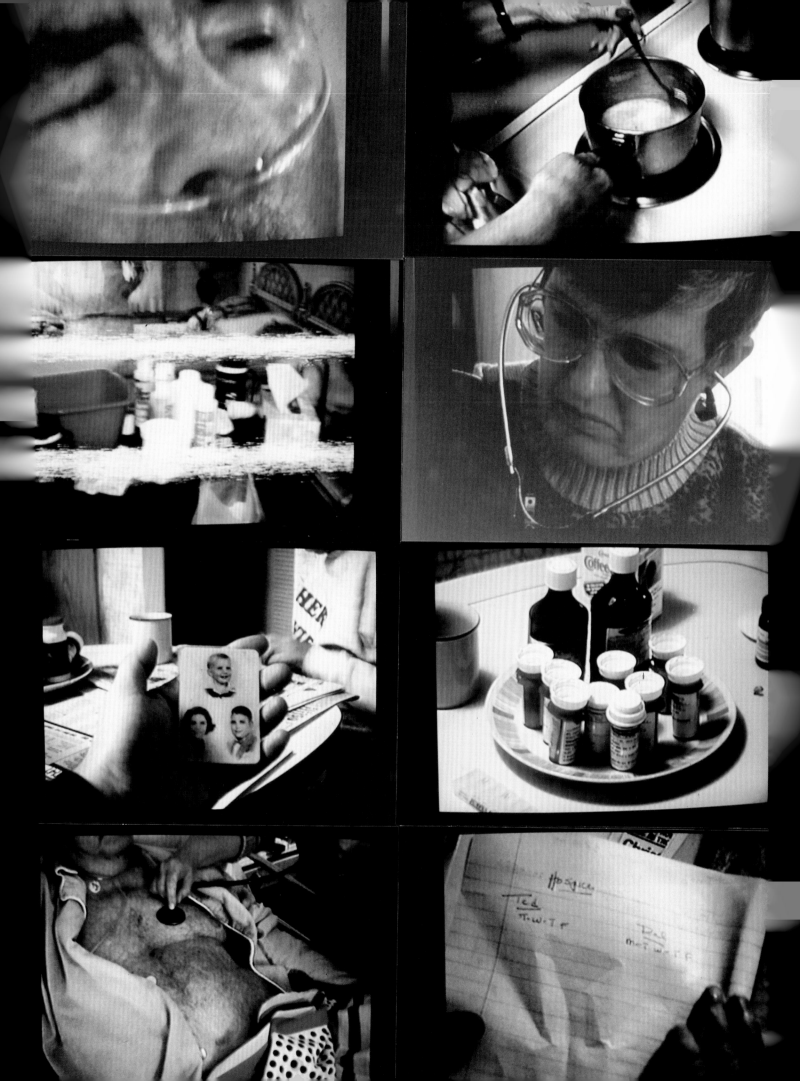

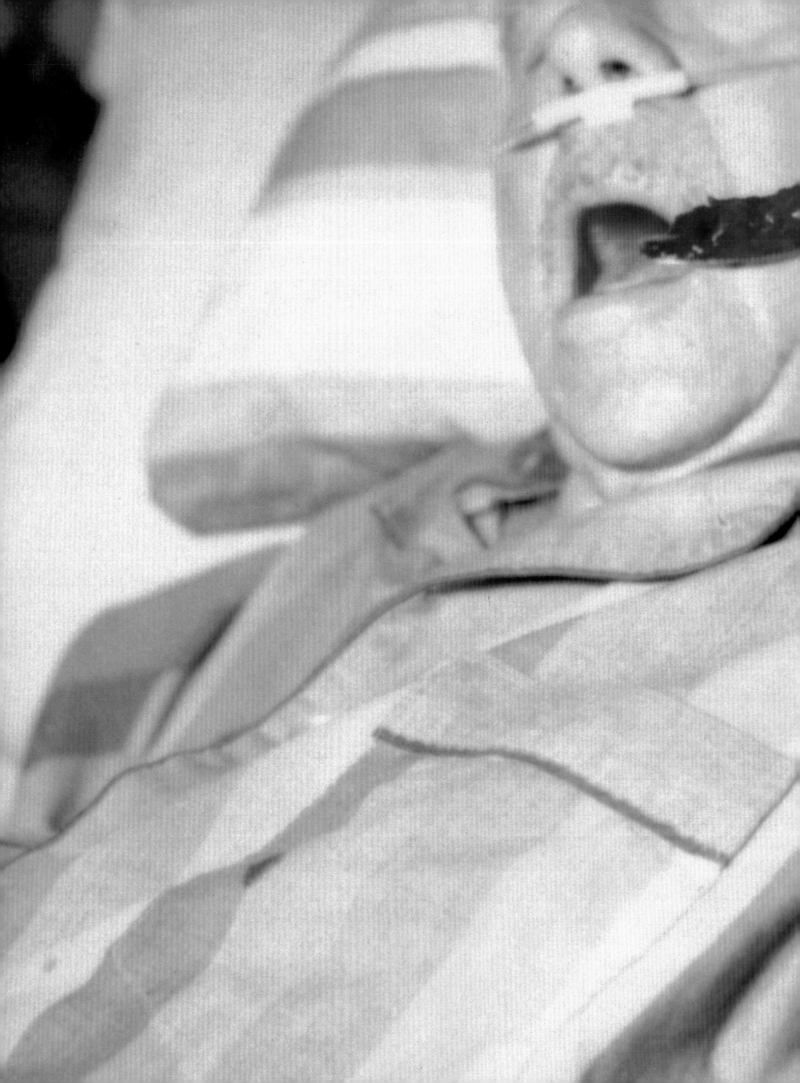

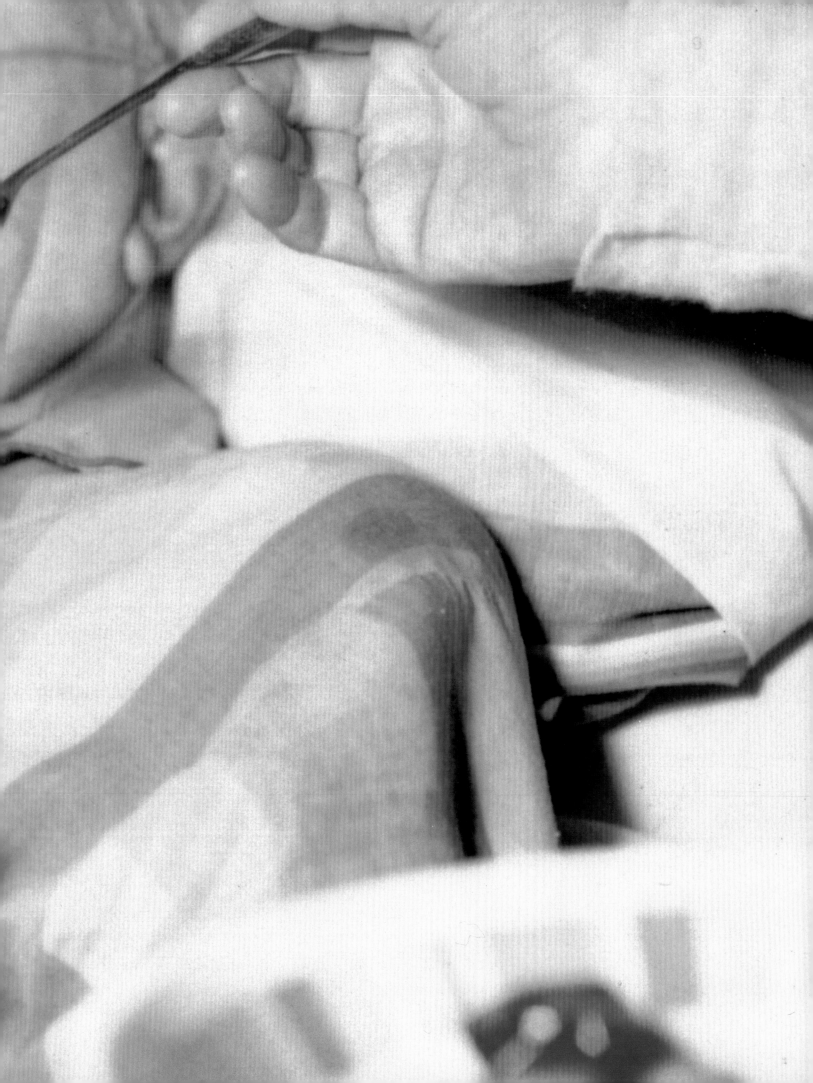

December 24 — Early Morning

I clasp my father, his body limp in my arms, and attempt to adjust his position. Perhaps he can be more comfortable and sleep. "I want my chair," he mumbles. He shuts his eyes. His breath is shallow and short. It's hard to tell if he's sleeping. His mouth is wide open, eyes half-shut. The oxygen machine drones.

It's the final round of *Wheel of Fortune.* The puzzle reads, T—E EN— —ONE. The clock is ticking. From somewhere in his unconscious mind Dad mutters, "The End Zone."

I move Mom's chair into their bedroom, next to my father's hospital bed. She sits and knits while Dad lies there tilted up in front of the large-screen TV. She is persistent in her attempts to comfort him. "Herb, darling, you can beat it," she says. She turns to me, stating, "Ever since your father had to get into this bed, he's let himself go downhill, thinking he's not going to make it." She turns back to him, leans close, and reiterates, "Sweetheart, you know you can do it, you've done it before. Do you want something to eat? I'm going to recharge the battery on your cart just in case you're feeling better. Okay, Goldie? You want to go for a ride?"

"Let me be," he blurts out.

Mom doesn't stop. She tells me about a dream he had last week, in which he hiked all the way to the county courthouse in Clearwater, screaming, "I can walk, I can walk!" When he woke up, he complained to Mom about pains in his legs. This is the first time I can remember that he can feel anything there. We give him Advil for the pain and Xanax to help him relax. We know he won't relax until we get him to his chair. Fran is out sick with the flu. No one from hospice can be here until tomorrow morning. I call the Utopia Home Care Agency. They agree to send Adam at eleven tonight. Mom isn't happy about "some stranger sleeping in my house."

pages 40–41
December 19, 1993 (Jell-o)

pages 44–45
Early That Morning, 1993

Christmas Eve, 1993

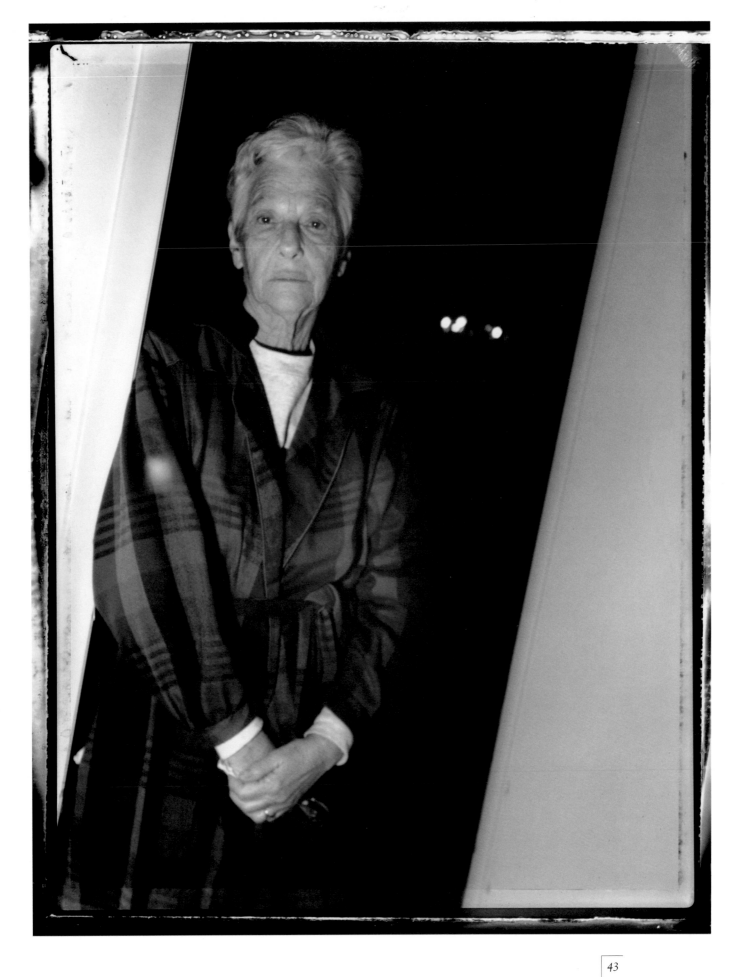

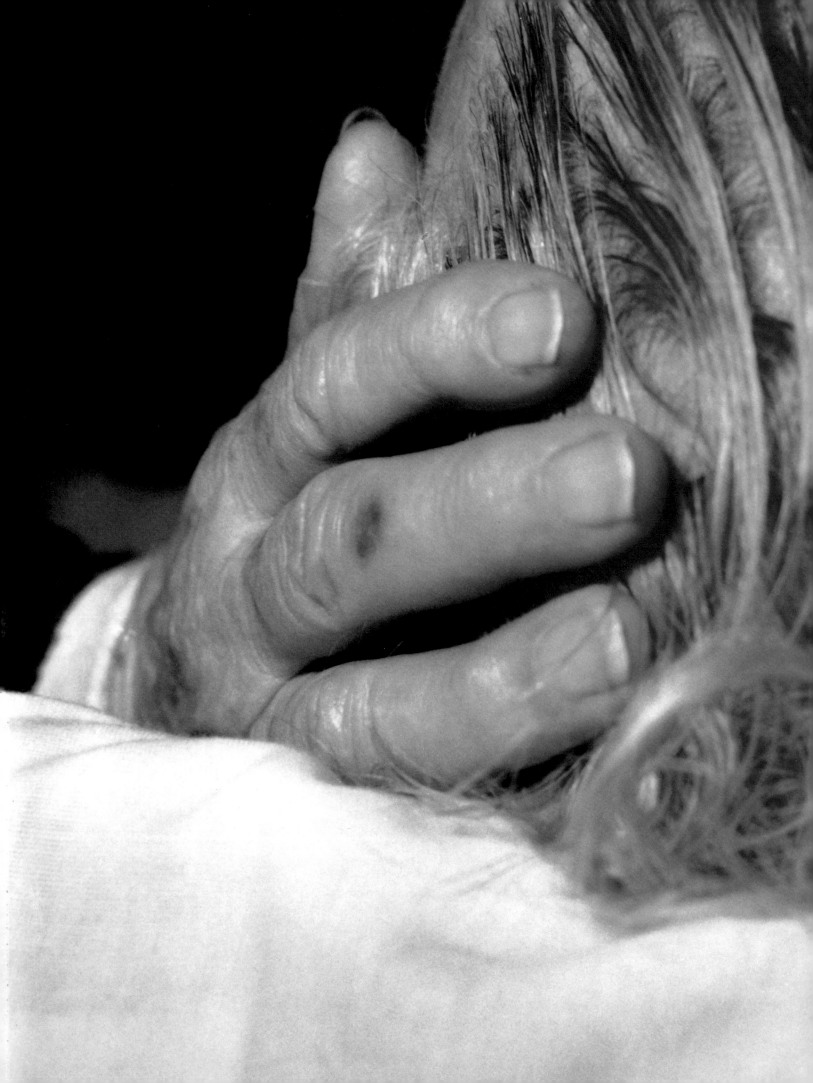

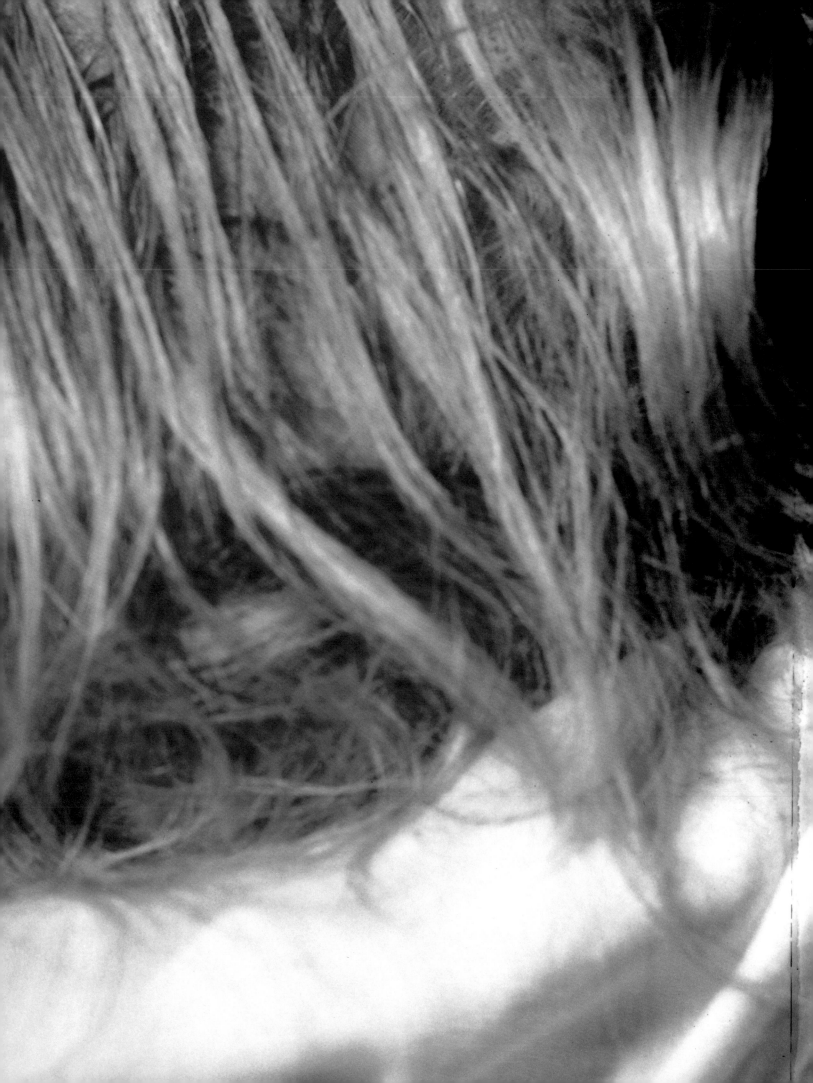

December 24 — Late Afternoon

Eyes shut, Dad's voice rises to a whisper: "Get me to my chair." My mother is hunched over Dad, singing a song from *Fiddler on the Roof* that they used to sing to each other: "Goldie, do you love me? Goldie? Do you love me?" His part is to answer, "Do I what?" but he doesn't.

The house is hot from the oxygen. A Polish woman comes to clean and vacuum the house. I step back for a moment to see what she sees here: the two of us scurrying around a sick man hidden away in a room, the door mostly closed. The feeling of death is everywhere.

Nighttime

It's raining. Melody Drive is a field of blurry Christmas lights. Cars filled with sightseeing old people — here to view the lights and get in the holiday spirit — roll by. I forget where I am for a moment.

Adam arrives. He is young, maybe nineteen, with lots of acne. His hair is short except for a tail hanging down his back. He wears a peace-sign earring and a Marlboro Gear T-shirt. Adam is introduced to Dad. My father shakes his head, indicating that he shat in his pants. Adam and I pull the sheet from underneath and carefully roll him to one side. Adam's pack of Marlboro Lights spills across the bed, cigarettes rolling between the sheets and my father's body. The diaper comes off and we find that Dad was mistaken. There is no mess. He expresses a fuzzy recognition that he has no idea what is going on. This is the moment I first see him lose control.

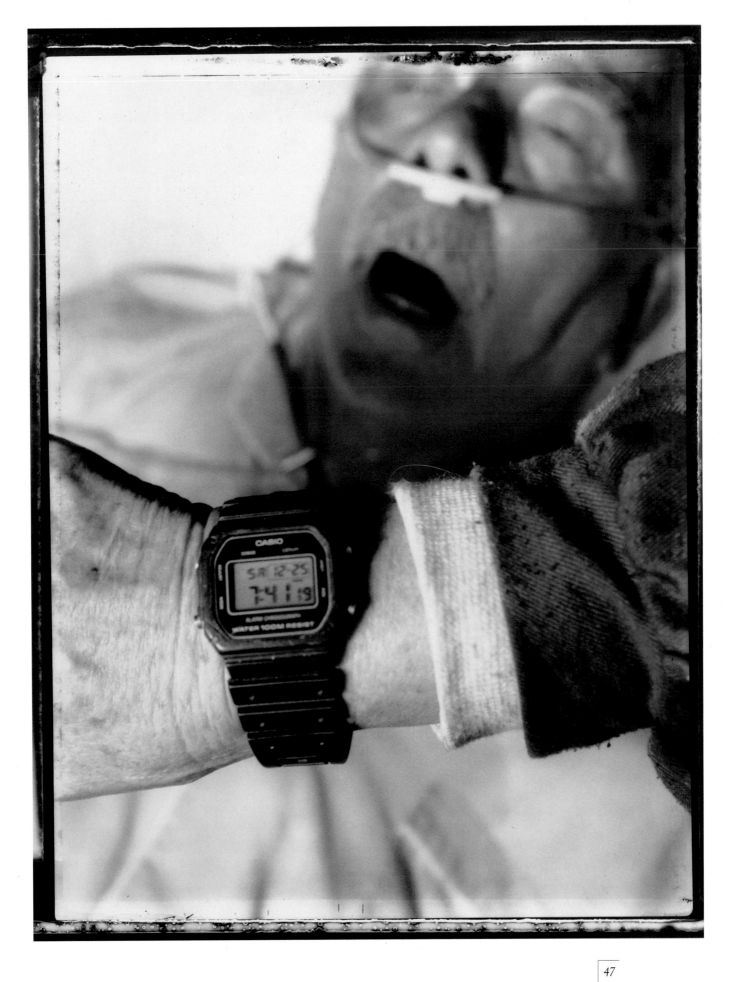

December 25 — 6:30 A.M.

There is an insecure tap, tap, tap on the door. "It's me, Adam. Your mom wants you to come out here, now." Mom is collapsed over Dad, crying and calling out, "I can't understand him. What do you want, Herb? Do you want me to raise the bed higher?"

Mom implores me to do something. "He's not breathing well. Can you help? Jimmy, you must help."
I move to Dad and put my ear to his lips. Faintly he says, "I can't breathe." I ask about the oxygen, and Adam says he tested it fifteen minutes ago. My father looks lunatic. I lean closer still and he says, "Say thank you." "To who, Dad?" I ask, going through the list of possibilities and finally arriving at Adam. Dad agrees with his eyes. Even in dying he is ever-graceful.

All of a sudden, with as much force as he can muster, Dad yells, "CHAIR!"

I ask Adam about his experience and his confidence wanes. Still, I'm determined to get Dad into his chair. I call hospice and leave a message for the Green Team nurse to call. I direct Mom to comfort Dad.

Mom begs, "Help him breathe, Jim."
I turn up the oxygen machine. Dad's eyes are glazed over. I tell him, "I'm right here, Dad."
"Chair," he whispers. The word is not quite discernible.
"I'm trying, Dad." I want to call Fran.
"No, it's Christmas and I don't want you to disturb anybody," Mom says. "It's not right."
"Mom, I don't know what's right now. I just know that he's dying and I've got to get him to his chair."
"Don't be so negative, Jimmy," she says. "Your father will make it. He always has." Mom kisses Dad while I photograph their last time together. It's an incredible stars-shining-in-your-eyes-as-tears-fall-down-on-us moment.

I see that Mom is about to offer coffee and cookies to Adam. He is nice, but I don't want him here now. "Not now, Mom," I declare. "We need to be alone with Dad." Adam leaves. I realize that all the things that my father couldn't be in his life don't matter now. I think that he's a strong, focused, great man. I must get him to his chair.

Time Speeds Up

Dad is losing consciousness, mumbling coma words. "What's he saying, Jim?" Mom asks.
"I don't know, Mom. Chair, I assume."
Hospice calls back. I describe how he can't breathe, and Rena, the nurse, says, "It sounds like the 'Death's Rattle.'" She tells me to rub Dad's hand and help him push forward, and that she'll check back in an hour.
I'm pleading to Dad, "Hold on till Fran gets here. Can you hear me?"
No more whispers.
No more breathing.
No more nothing.

7:41 A.M.

He is dead. My mom is begging me to give him more oxygen. I explain it won't help. Hospice calls. Someone will be over in thirty minutes. Mom is crying and goes out to get the paper. She comes back in. It's a beautiful, clear, cold morning. The headlines read, FLORIDA GETS A WINTRY SLAP FOR THE HOLIDAY and BETHLEHEM CHRISTMAS IS JOYOUS AND POLITICAL. The house is still warm from the oxygen. Dad is now cold.

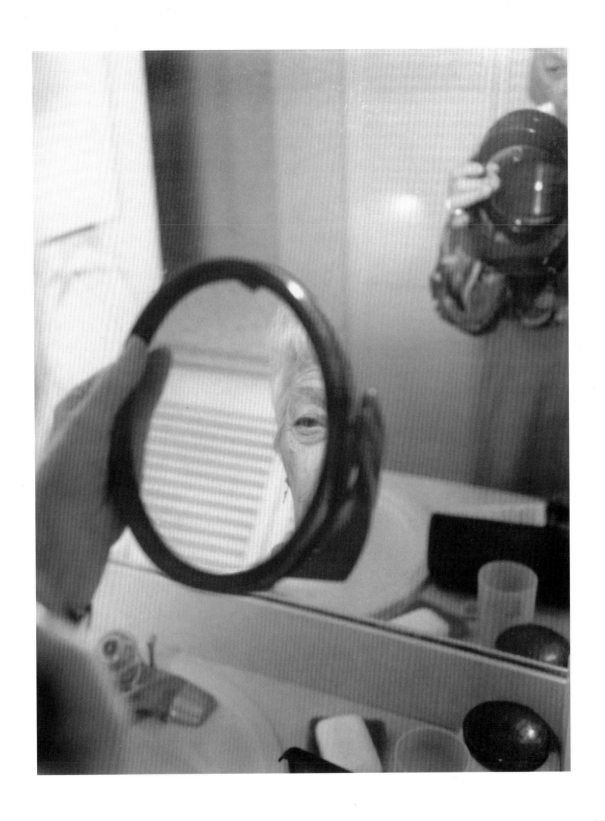

*Mom Getting Ready for
the Funeral,* 1993

pages 50–51
*Melody Drive,
Palm Harbor, Florida,* 1993

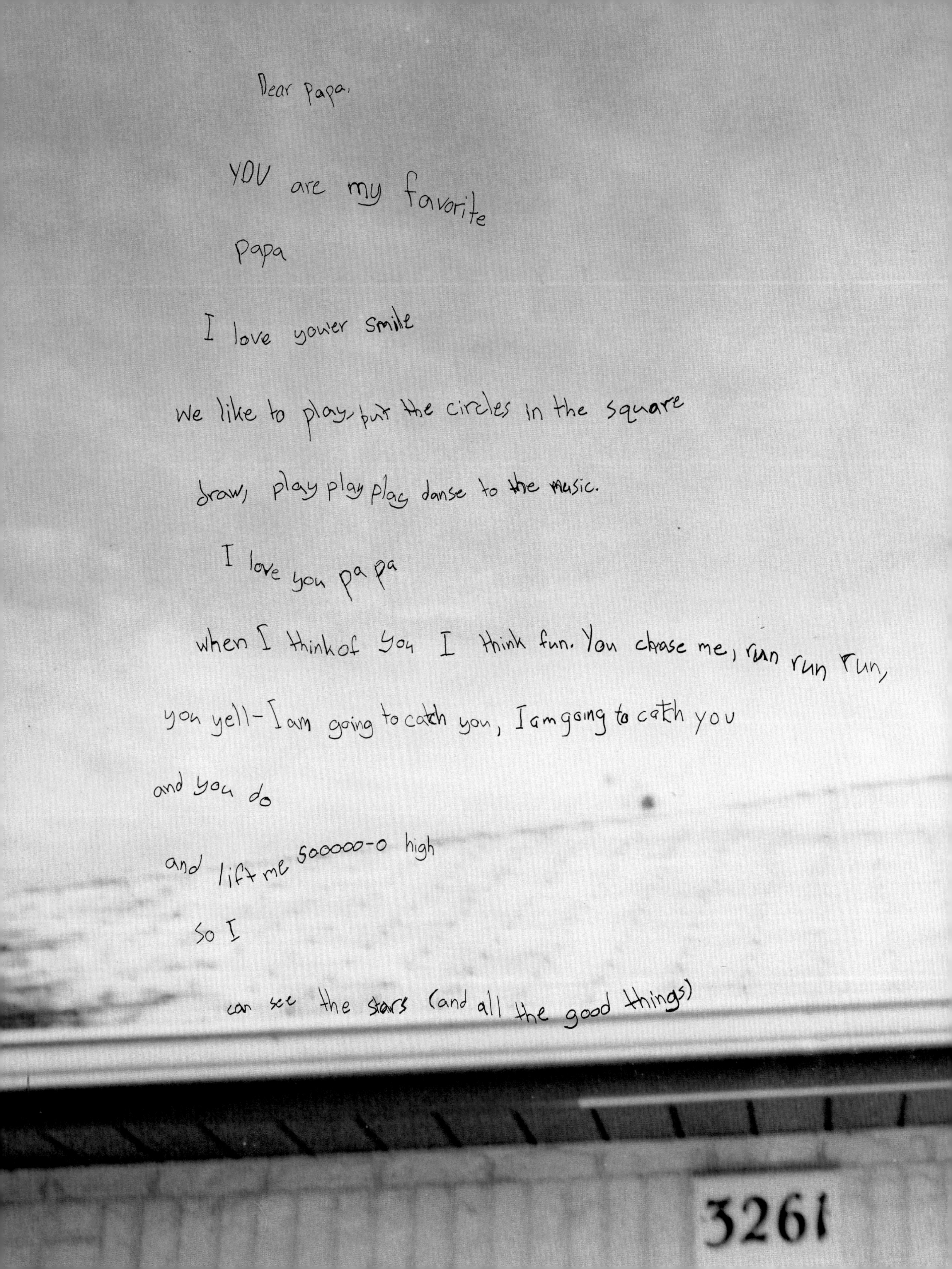

Dear Papa,

YOU are my favorite
Papa

I love yower smile

We like to play, put the circles in the square

draw, play play play danse to the music.

I love you pa pa

when I think of you I think fun. You chase me, run run run,

you yell—I am going to catch you, I am going to catch you

and you do

and lift me sooooo-o high

So I

can see the stars (and all the good things)

3261

lie down all tired
crickets at night are pretty
see the night,

nighty, night

I dreem I am out in the grass, running down the hills so fast
so fast
and I fall and cry
I wake up in my bed so sad papa
because I get so lonely

I wish that you and Mama sleep with me

But you come to me in my eyes

then I sleep. dont wake up and cry now.

I am happy

You are my only PaPa

I dreem my Mommy and Daddy.

NAN GOLDIN

Philip Brookman: What brought you to work with the people that you did?

Nan Goldin: I worked with the Cabrini Hospice in New York City. I photographed people with AIDS because, with the illnesses and deaths of so many of my friends, that's what I've been close to in my own life for the past dozen years. I also photographed people with other illnesses. I made repeated visits to most of the people and tried to photograph them with lovers, spouses, siblings, and children.

PB: What did you set out to accomplish?

NG: I needed to face my own denial of death and learn more about how people come to accept mortality. I wanted to document — as much as possible — the complexity of the people I photographed and the interiors of the spaces they lived in. I was interested in how their environments affected and reflected their mood, and what objects and places became important to them. I wanted to make more than a one-dimensional portrait of the different patients, to capture their moments of pleasure and anger, their ambivalence about their lives, and their approaching deaths.

PB: What unique experiences did you have?

NG: It was fascinating to see the differences in each person's acceptance of death and the roles that human love, spiritual belief, and humor play in this process. I realized that the only thing that separates me from the dying is time.

PB: How was this project different from your previous work?

NG: This project was also motivated by my obsession with recording my life and the lives of my friends. It was about making amends to those who had died when I hadn't been there. Two of my closest friends, Cookie Mueller and Vittorio Scarpati, died as in-patients at Cabrini Hospice in 1989. I wasn't there and I had no clear concept of what a hospice was, so I wanted to learn where they had been and what they'd gone through. That's why I

was interested in Cabrini. When I began this work, I had just returned from Europe, where I had witnessed two other close friends become ill and die. After photographing their deaths I couldn't take a picture for a long time. I was no longer so afraid to confront illness or death, however, so I shared some of my experiences with the people I visited for hospice. Everyone I met touched me, and a few people I grew to care for deeply. This process allowed me to confront feelings that were too close and too painful to face before.

PB: Has your understanding of the hospice concept changed?

NG: I was not very familiar with hospice. After getting to know it a little I was very impressed by the people and their philosophy. Some members of communities heavily affected by AIDS have been put off by hospice because so many people with AIDS are ill at a premature point in their lives. Their emphasis is on living rather than dying. But having watched the treatment some friends have received in New York hospitals, I think that hospice is a vital option. In America, hospice care — the process of helping patients and survivors face their impending loss, controlling pain, enabling patients to get their lives in order, and bereavement counseling — is essential. I learned this after watching how hard it is for people to die without this kind of assistance and comfort.

PB: Has your understanding of photography changed?

NG: Photographing people in hospice care — looking at suffering and grace in strangers' lives — expanded my interest in documenting emotional worlds outside my own. This enabled me to see that there can be a meaningful relationship between photographer and subject that develops between strangers, given a degree of empathy. I'm addicted to photographing the most intense periods in our lives. During my project, I sometimes felt that connection with people at an essential point in their lives.

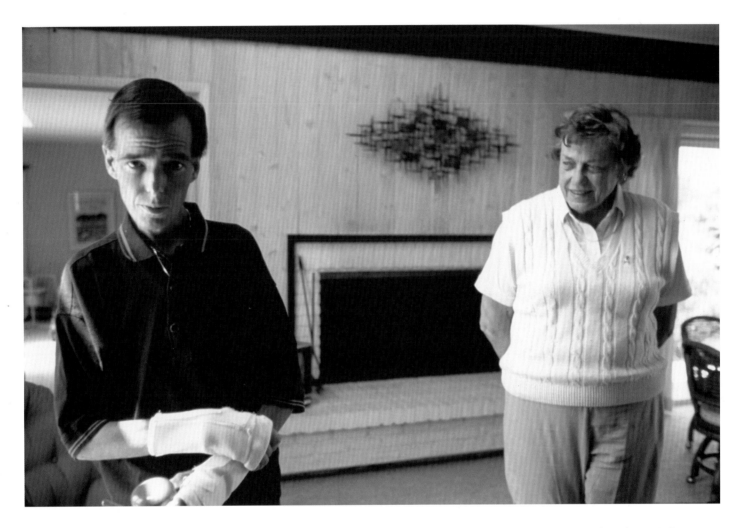

PB: Is it possible to photograph the passing of life?

NG: For me, the only subject in photography is the recording of life and its passage. I think that's why photography was invented. Some of the earliest photographs were deathbed daguerreotypes. I used to think that if I photographed a person enough, I would never lose them. With the deaths of so many friends, I've learned the limitation of the medium. In spite of my frustration—this crisis of belief—I still feel that pictures of people ensure their continued presence on some level, and that it's important to make traces of a person's life as a form of homage. For me, photography has always been about staving off loss. My pictures help me remember how much I've lost.

Bucky with His Mother,
Quogue, New York, 1995

53

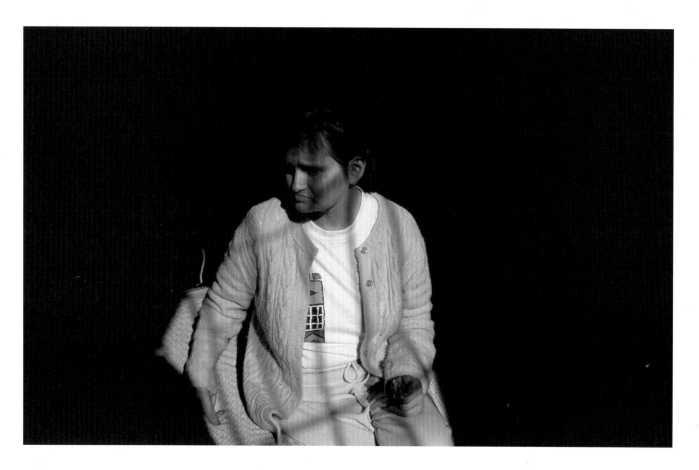

Carmen at Home,
New York City, 1994

upper right
Carmen's Medicine,
New York City, 1994

lower right
Carmen with Poppi,
New York City, 1994

pages 56–57
Carmen with Jonathan and Gloria,
New York City, 1994

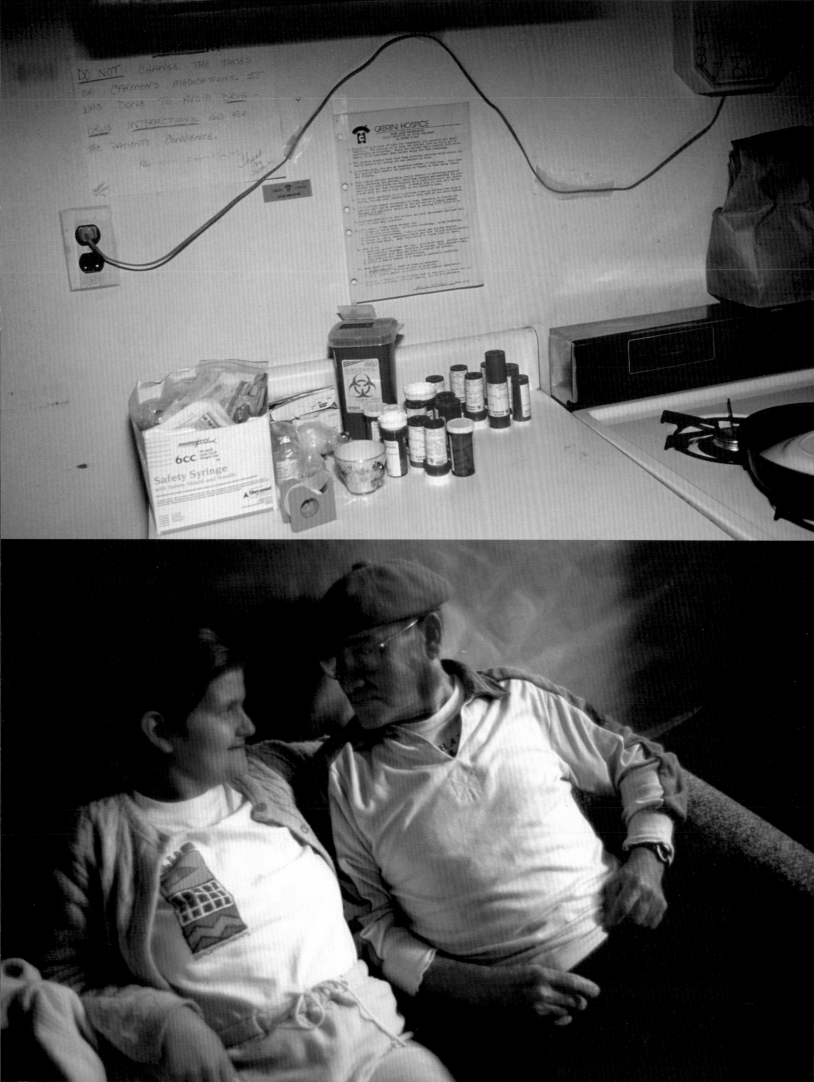

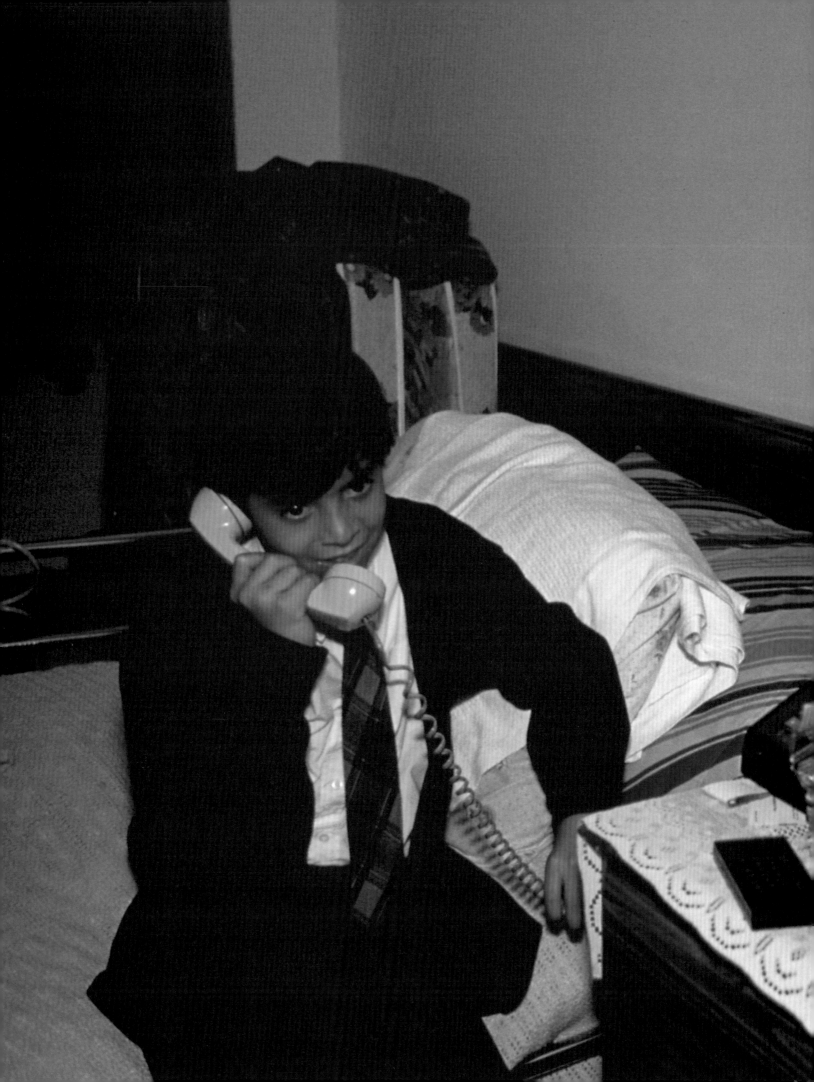

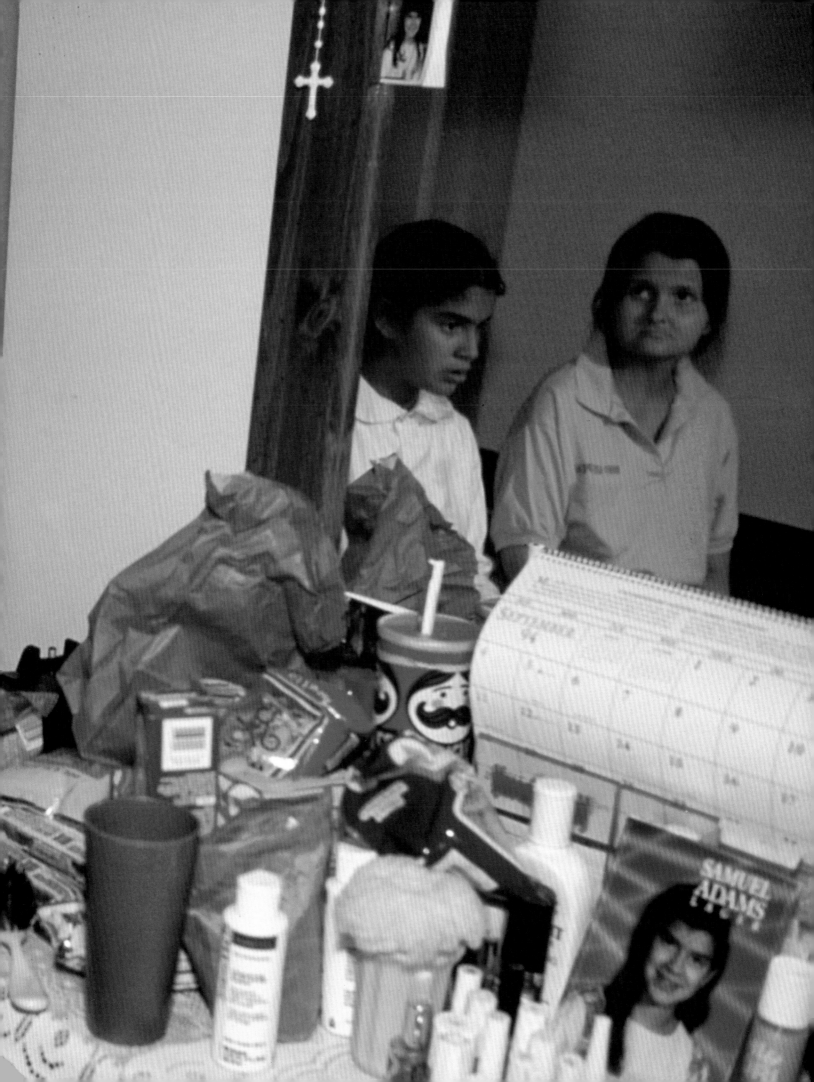

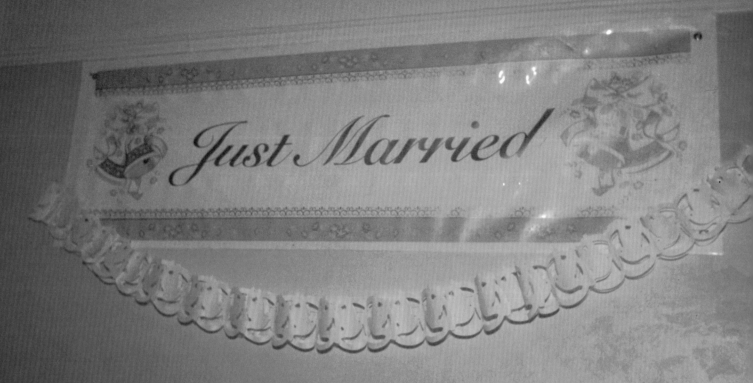

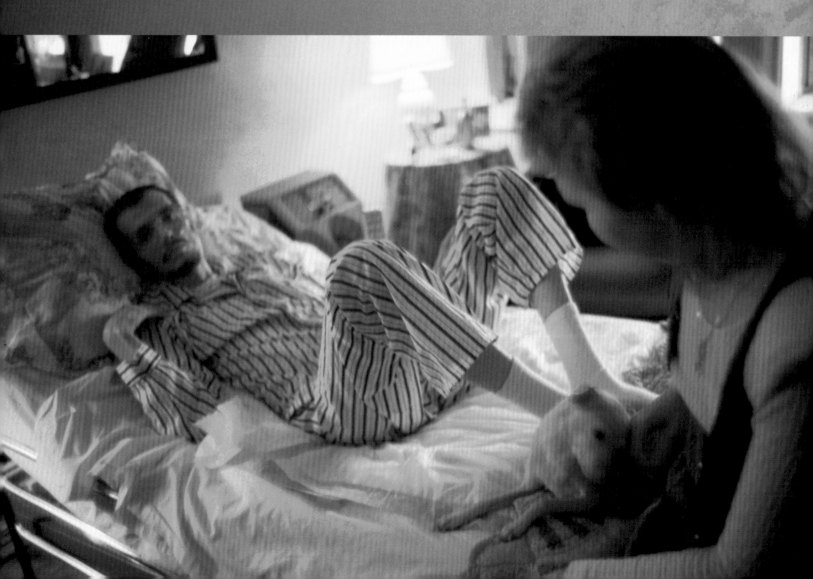

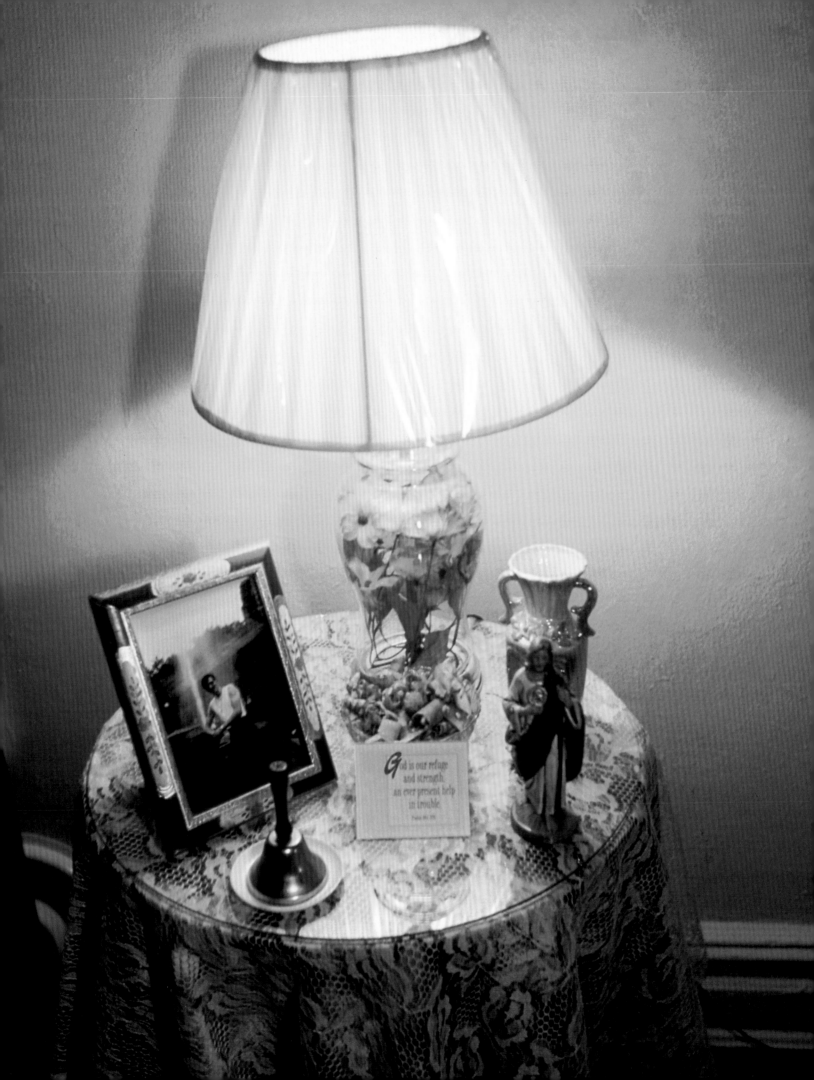

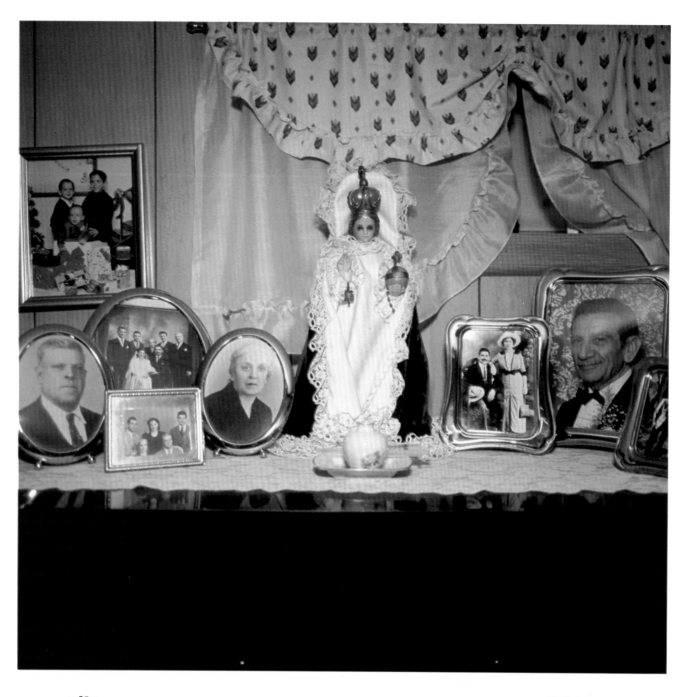

page 58, top
Just Married,
New York City, 1995

page 58, bottom
Larry and Margot at Home,
New York City, 1995

page 59
Larry's Table,
New York City, 1995

Emilia's Dresser, Brooklyn
1994

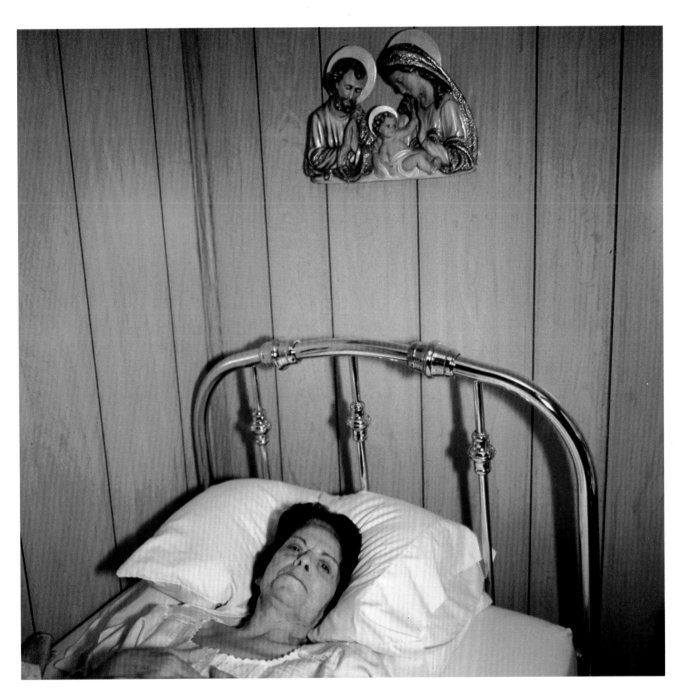

Emilia, Brooklyn
1994

Grace, a former hospice worker, could hardly hold her head up because of brain cancer. But she was still so concerned about the needs of her husband. He was partially deaf and she was going blind, so they'd become symbiotic: she was his ears and he was her eyes. She was deeply religious and spiritual; their son, who'd been a priest, had come to take care of her. She talked openly about her death.

Bucky, who was in the final stages of AIDS and in a lot of pain, was still so eager to make me comfortable. He was full of grace and humor. He was thrilled about the exhibition because he'd gone to the Corcoran School of Art years ago. His mother, who'd adopted him as an infant, stood strong beside him. Her husband had died a year before in hospice. Bucky's longtime lover had died a year or two before. He'd lived a long time with the illness. He died soon after my visit.

Carmen had the love and care of a much older husband, Poppi, who also had AIDS, but she was very depressed and spent most of her time watching television and eating candy. Her house was dark and the visiting nurse (not from hospice) gave us "Watchtower" literature and was AIDSphobic — she always wore rubber gloves. Carmen's children, who were in foster care, visited once a week.

Larry had given up — he seemed isolated on his bed, except for his wife and dog. The house was full of his wife's drawings and *chatchkes.* They'd recently been married. She'd worked as a bartender in a bar in Times Square very much like the one I worked in from 1980 to 1985, and Larry was one of the neighborhood guys who'd frequented the bar. She seemed to be his only remaining connection to the world.

Emilia was first-generation Sicilian. Her daughter, Jenny, lived in a little suburban Italian enclave of Brooklyn and had set up the basement in the house for her mother, where she took devoted, constant care of her. Jenny's beautiful sons were close to their grandmother, and Emilia was dying in the context of a loving family. She had Jenny do her makeup when I came to photograph.

I first met Joseph when he was in Cabrini Hospice and later at his Chelsea apartment. Joseph is angry, and I think his anger has kept him alive. I videotaped him for a BBC documentary, and the BBC also came and did a shoot of us together. He said the documentary gave him something to look forward to, as he wanted to speak out about AIDS from his experience, to help other people. He'd worked as a blackjack dealer in Atlantic City and longed to go back near the ocean. He'd also been homeless in New York for two years until he went to work for Housing Works — an AIDS service organization that runs a thrift shop. He had a vivid repertoire of stories from the various lives he'd lived. He'd modeled a little, and was interested in working for a modeling agency that uses people with AIDS as models. He played me the Shirley Horn song, "Here's to Life," and held my hand and wept. We got him hooked up with John Giorno's AIDS project, which sends money directly to people with AIDS. My assistants and I brought him food and watched talk shows with him.

Amalia's *joie de vivre* was a real revelation to us; she was so full of life and humor, and surrounded by the love of a household full of women. Her mother had moved back to New York from Puerto Rico to take care of her, and her older daughters had come back from college. She had numerous siblings and two little girls. I envied the love in that family — I teased them that I was going to move in. Amalia told us great stories; emaciated from cancer, she scared the neighborhood kids by making herself up like a ghoul and answering the door on Halloween. Her environment, with all its color and playful detail, was in sharp contrast to Carmen's and undoubtedly contributed to her living much longer than expected.

I felt that Joseph, Amalia, and Bucky were people I would have become friends with in my own life; we shared a language. But I also learned a lot from people I wouldn't have usually come into contact with, about a wider commonality of experience that I didn't know existed.

Nan Goldin

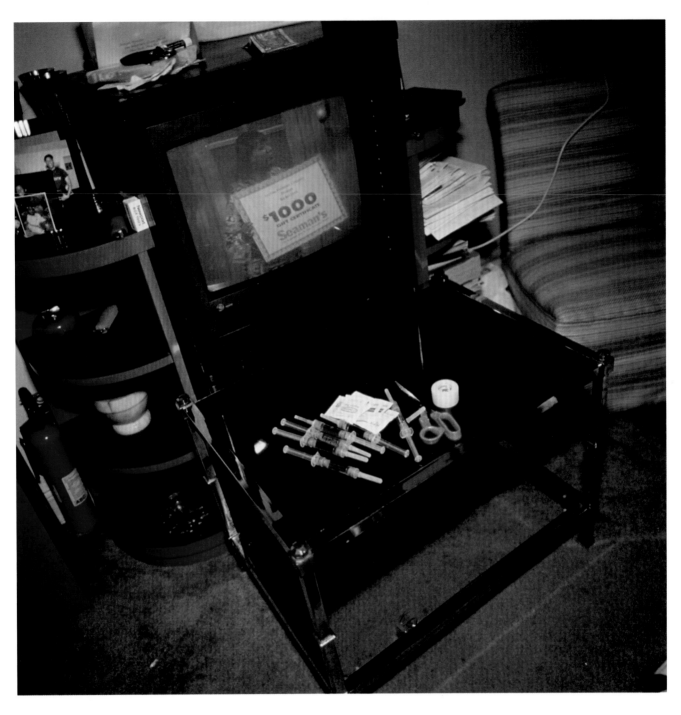

Joseph's Medicine,
New York City, 1995

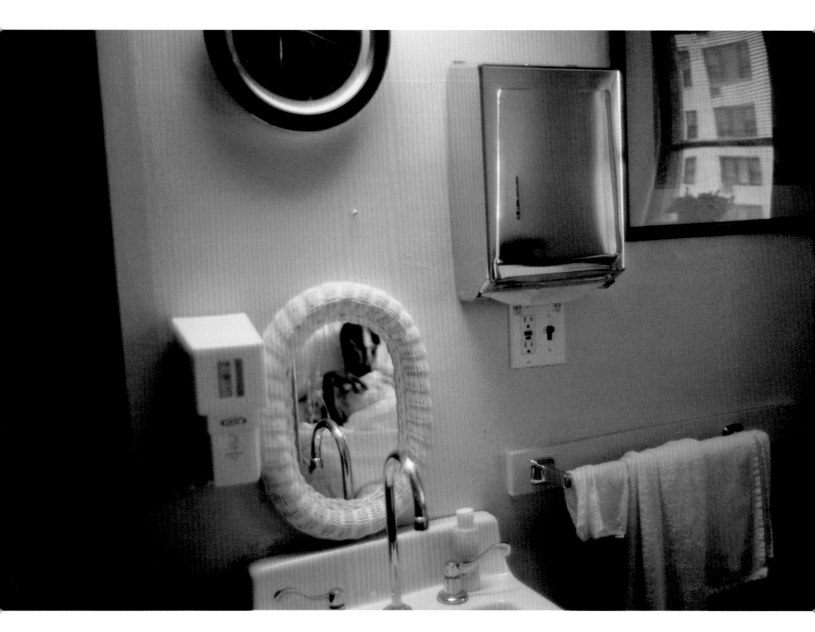

Joseph at Cabrini Hospice,
New York City, 1995

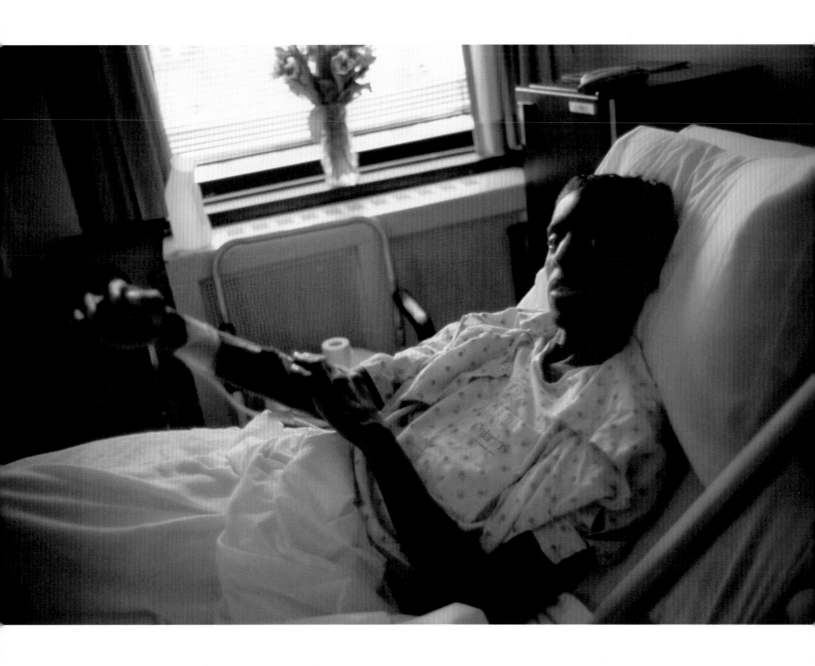

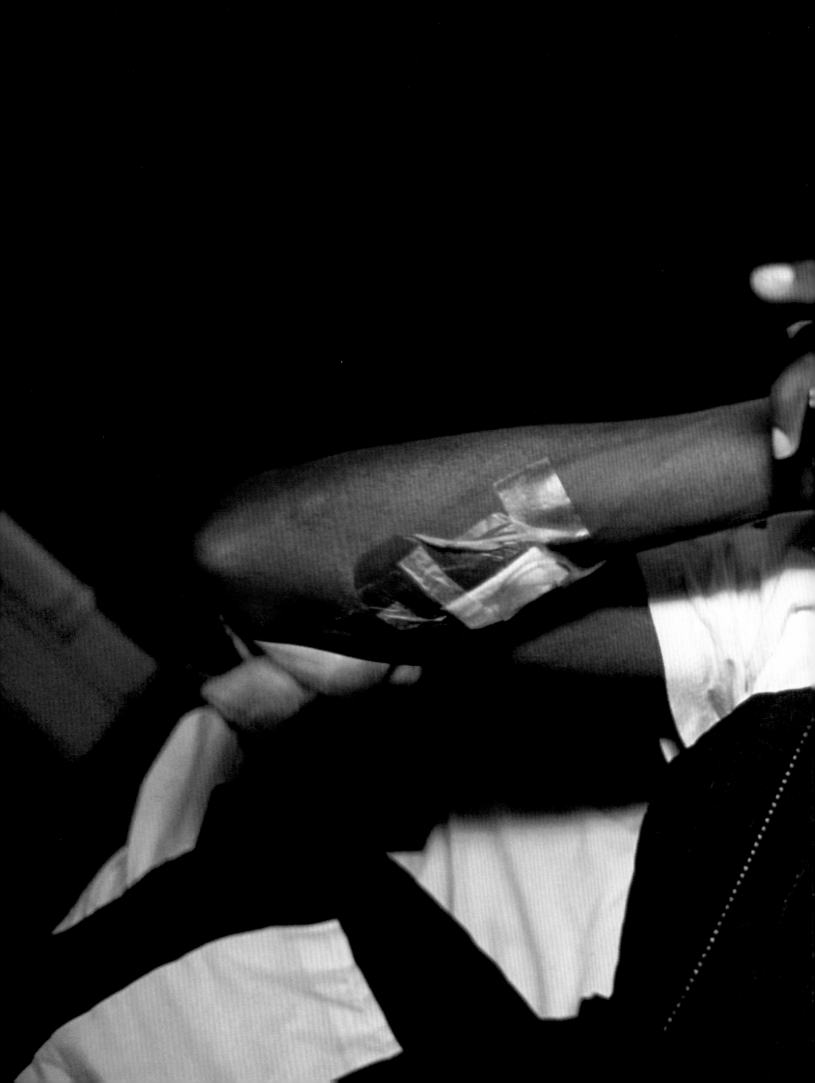

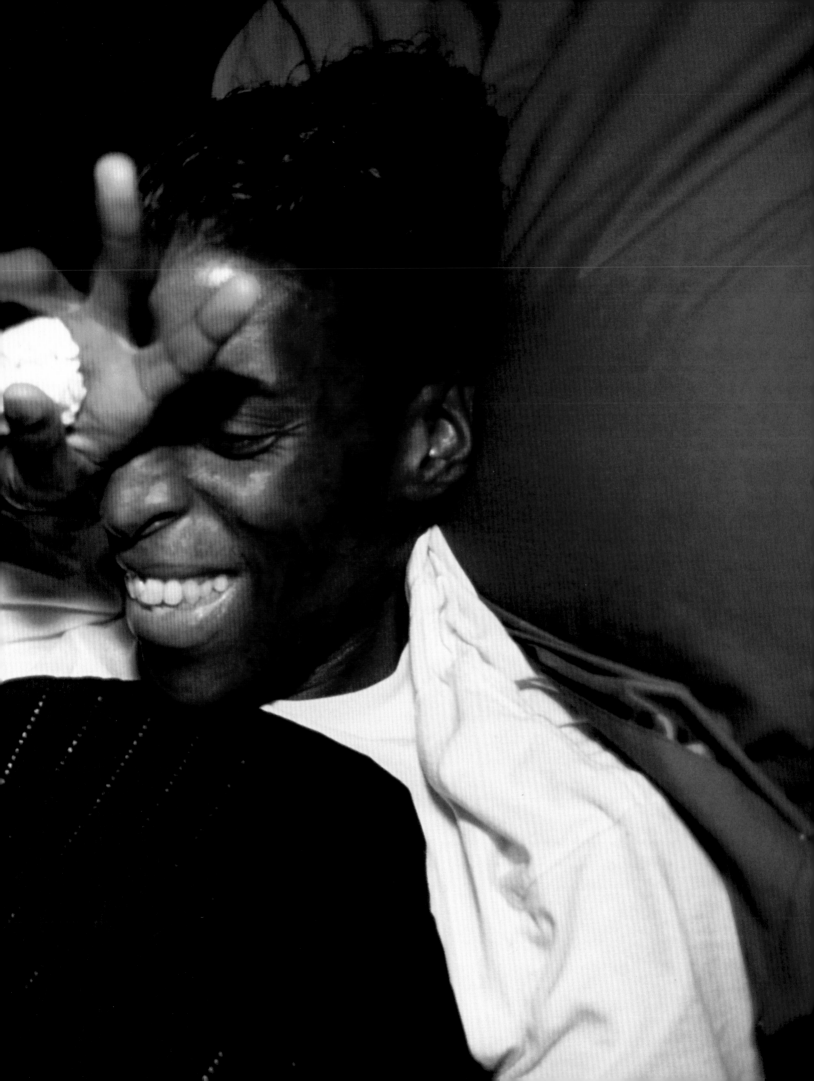

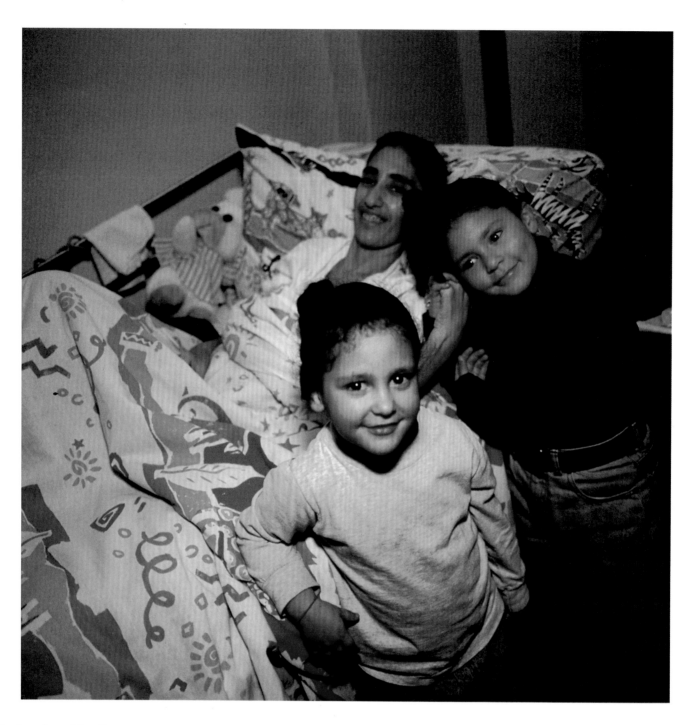

Amalia, Amanda, and Jennifer,
New York City, 1994

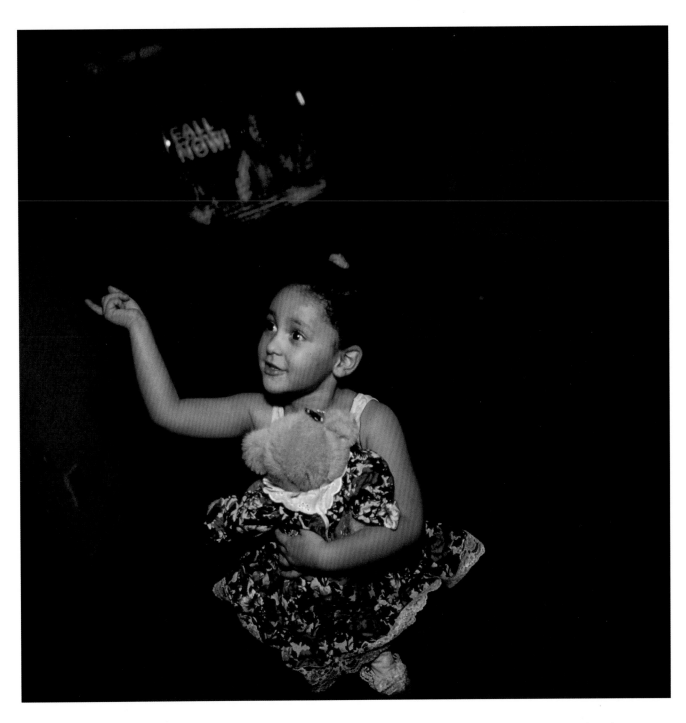

Amanda,
New York City, 1994

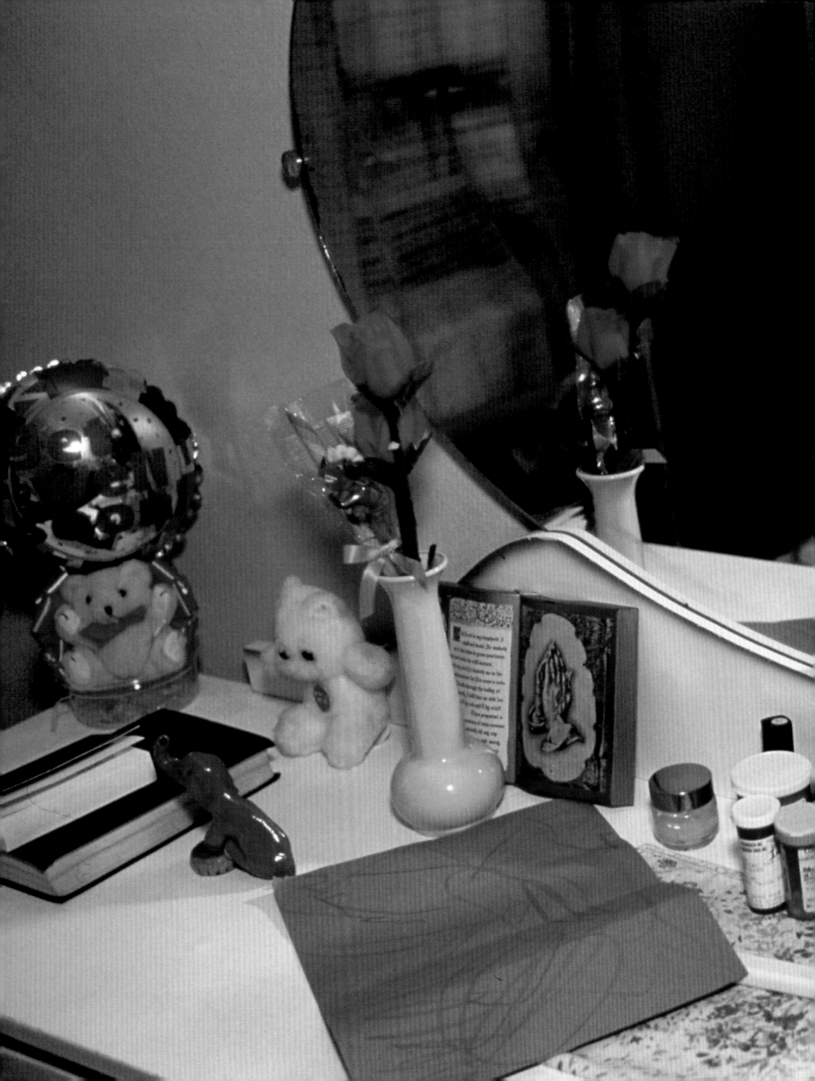

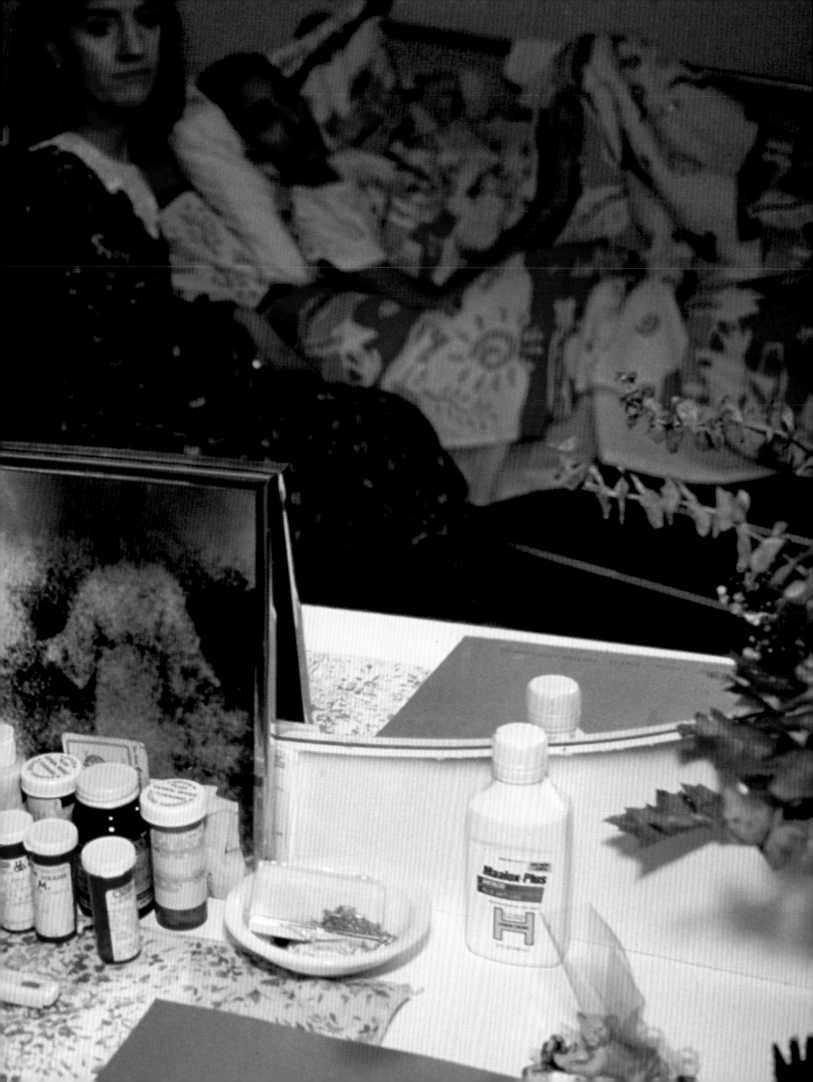

pages 70–71
Amalia's Dresser,
New York City, 1994

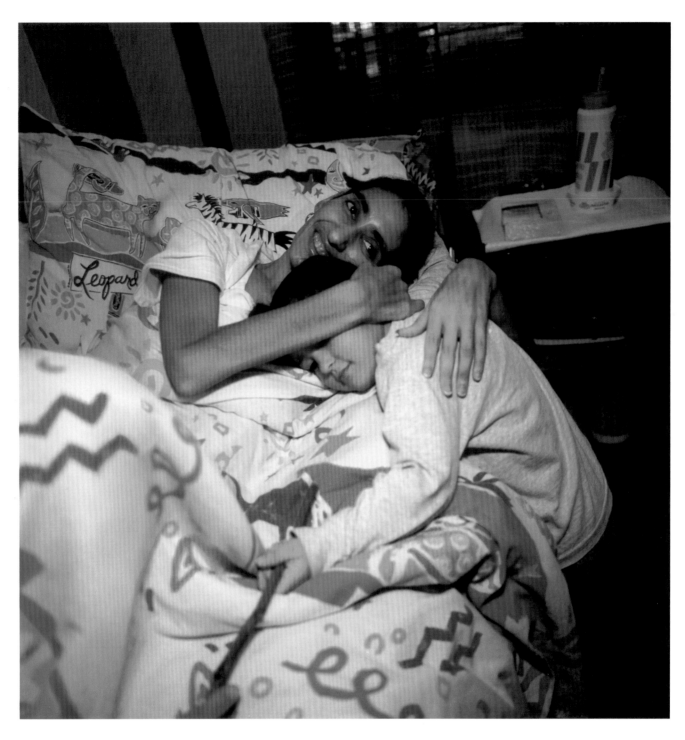

Amalia and Amanda,
New York City, 1994

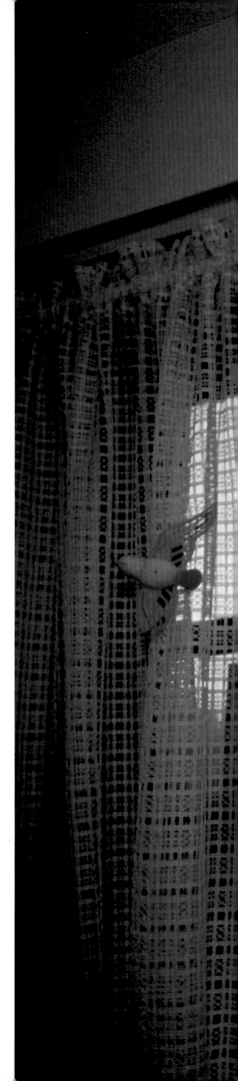

Curtain in Amalia's Room,
New York City, 1994

74

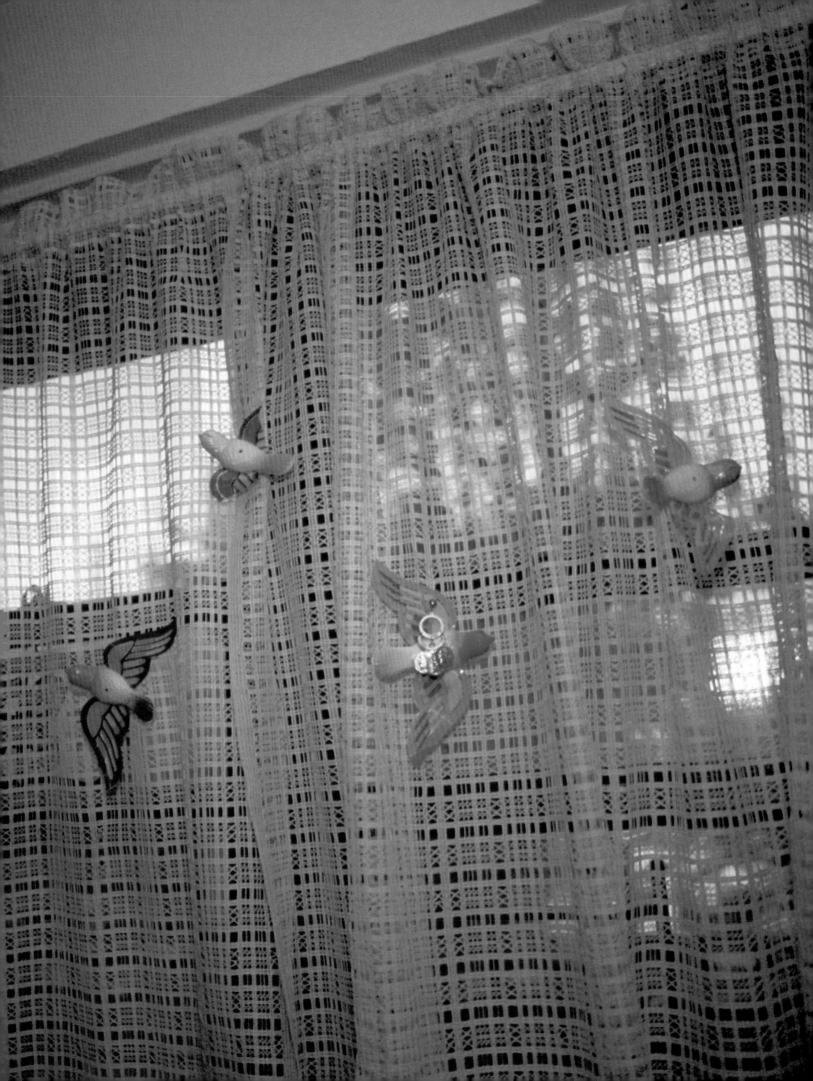

SALLY MANN

Philip Brookman: Where did you photograph and what brought you to work at these places and with the people that you did?

Sally Mann: I felt that the hospice photographs should be made here in Lexington, the community where I live and work. By happy coincidence, one of my best friends, Joan Robins, is a hospice nurse here. Joan had cared for my father in his last months and is familiar with my approach to making photographs. I went with her when she visited patients. In the beginning we were concerned that having me along might compromise her relationship with them, but we found that not to be the case.

PB: These photographs, combined with your words, are like a meditation on life and death in a small Southern town. What did you set out to accomplish with this project and how did you develop it?

SM: While watching Joan interact with her patients, I hoped to discover something universal about how we approach death. I was in search of what exactly it is that *matters* to the dying person and how hospice tries to provide those things. This question — of ultimate desire — has interested me for a long time. In the same way that my children ask, "What would you take out of the house if it were on fire?" I wondered whether the trivial or the transcendent assumes greater importance in our final months. I suspected it might be the former, just as my own answer to the fire question is never "my art" but always "the scrapbooks."

PB: What unique experiences did you have working with Joan?

SM: My encounters with patients in their homes were as varied and fascinating as humanity itself. There was a wealth of heartbreakingly gay, poignant, and absurd material at each stop. But most remarkable to me was how the presence of death seemed to make unnecessary the reserve and distrust with which strangers to the home are often greeted. At each door, Joan, of course, was greeted warmly. But I, a stranger with a camera, was welcomed no less warmly.

PB: Much of your work has been about your own life and environs, your family, and those around you. How is this project different from your previous work?

SM: Speaking technically, I chose a greater depth of field than I have in my earlier photographs because, for the hospice work, I thought details were more important than ambience. I wanted more of the image to be in focus. Obviously, I am somewhat more removed, more the objective observer than I am in the work with my family.

PB: Is it possible to record something as abstract and temporal as the passing of life?

SM: There is a picture in the book *Gramp* which comes as close to catching the actual moment of death as any I have ever seen. In it, the dying man raises an emaciated arm, fist clenched, in a gesture that resembles one made in defiance. Because of the vitality of the gesture, there is no way to know that this man is drawing his last breath. Similarly, there are few clues to inform the casual observer that the man I photographed stretched out on the couch in his bathrobe — my father — is similarly lifeless. By the time the breath actually leaves the body, the experience of dying has already occurred. Photography can capture aspects of that experience which, taken together, can help us understand the passage of life. My pictures are about trying to discover the *vincula,* the ties that bind.

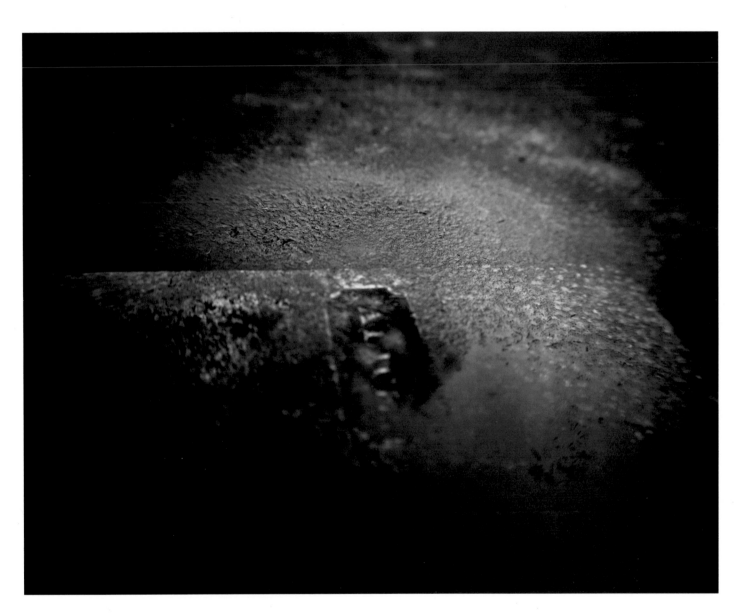

Paradoxically, patients often ask to visit the grave sites of family and friends.

Windows

The sick person's best medicine is desire. . . . When I was in the hospital, I was always gazing out of the window at the real world, which had never looked more desirable. I'd like to suggest . . . keeping one's desire alive as a way of keeping oneself alive.

Anatole Broyard, *Intoxicated by My Illness*

What patients see from their windows becomes vital to them. Hospice workers stress the importance of moving patients to allow them a view outside, even if it means a major disruption of the medical set-up. When they look out, the scene is often unprepossessing, the objects in their view random and unaffecting. The old bucket, the dog sprawled under the eaves, become touchstones, become their very world.

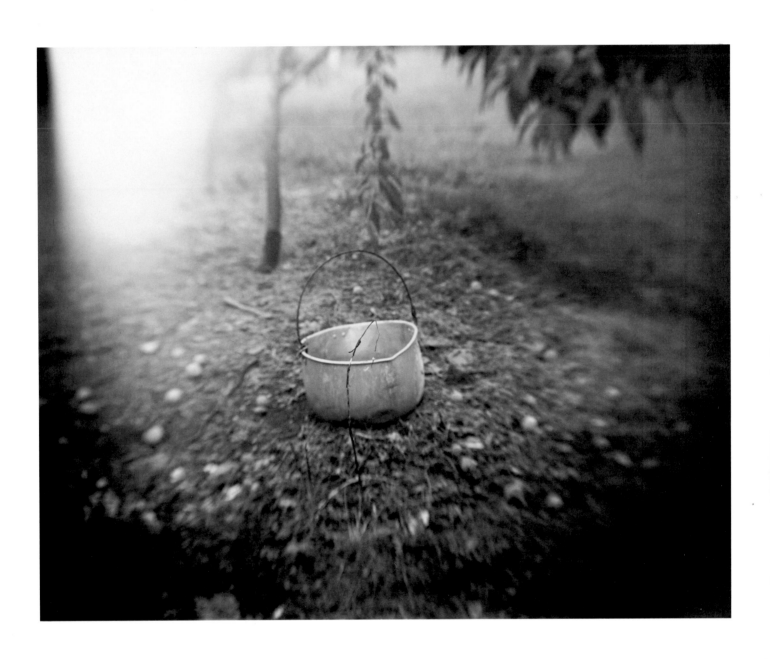

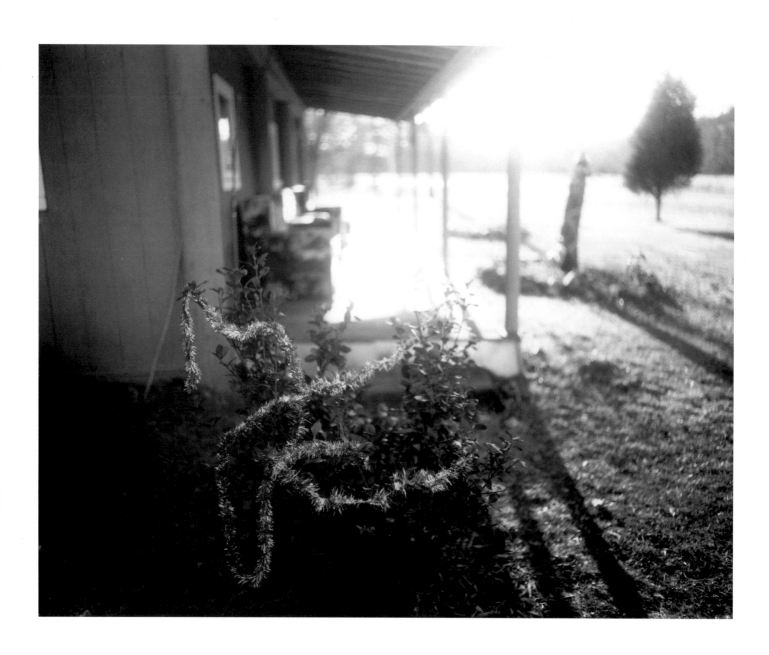

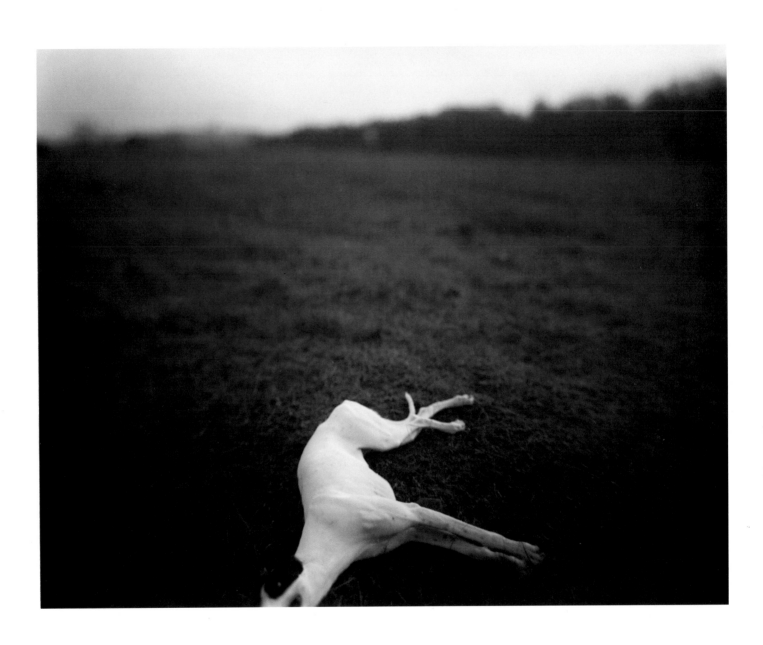

Joan's Patients

On my first trip with Joan, we drove toward Glasgow to a smallish, neat house set in a cleared area. This house belonged to the daughter of the dying woman. Sleeping on a fold-out couch in the living room, the daughter had moved her mother into her own bedroom as the illness progressed. This was where we headed.

In the large bed was a slight, S-shaped wrinkle. It looked like the kind of ripple that remains after the covers have been thrown back over a vacated bed. The patient was tiny in all her features, except one hand that had swollen to monstrous proportions, basketball-sized. It was so saturated with fluid that it wept on the sheets. Her sparse white hair was splayed out on the pillow as if it were waving.

Behind her was a painting of the classic Indian maiden, robust and defiant, her hair streaming back in the unseen wind in painful mimicry of the white hair on the pillow below. She was perfect in all her parts, and her muscular arm held a bow at the ready.

Stupidly, I began to cry. Joan shot nervous glances at me. I left the room. Dispirited, I photographed the window at which, in better health, the patient had sat and worked on her quilts.

When the daughter came out, I mentioned the painting. She said there used to be many paintings of Indians in the bedroom, but her mother had asked that all but that one be taken out. The daughter said her mother didn't really like Indians all that much; they were too violent.

On the way back I thought about how I felt about this stranger, this wrinkle in the covers who'd made me cry. I thought about how we assign higher virtues to the dying person, how I thought of her more tenderly than I might have if she had been a gum-smacking, cranky, ambulatory old lady. Probably I wouldn't have had much in common with this woman; certainly our attitudes toward Native Americans diverged. Yet seeing her so helpless and reduced brought out a flood of irrational affection.

I felt a similar emotion that night, looking at a picture of the big-eared, withered old man being retried for the murder of Medgar Evers. I was confused by the protective feelings roused by this white supremacist who managed to offend me on several different levels when he allowed this curious opinion: "Killing that nigger gave me no more inner discomfort than our wives endure when they give birth to our children."

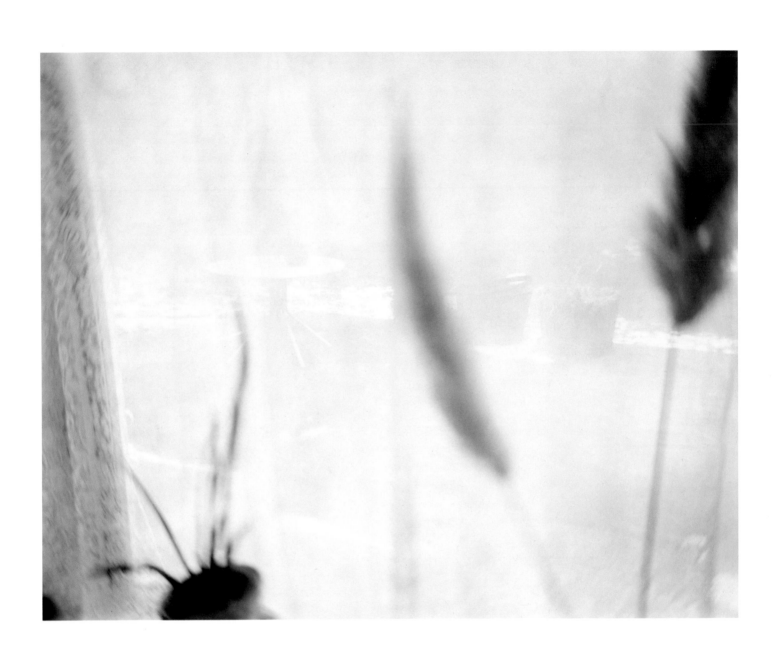

When did you last see your father? *I try to remember where I first heard the question asked, or saw it written. I invent contexts for it. . . . When did you last see your father? A friend says: "You know it's a painting, of course. . . . It hung on the stairs in my boarding-school, the first thing you'd see each term, just what you needed when your father had dumped you like a sack of potatoes. You know the one — it's incredibly famous." I don't know it, or if I do I've forgotten. But suddenly everybody I meet seems to allude to it, or parody the phrase. . . . I turn up the painting shortly afterwards . . . a Cavalier boy standing stiffly on a stool before a table of Puritan inquisitors — "And When Did You Last See Your Father?" I suppose I must have seen the painting before, but if so I'd forgotten it. Certainly I'd forgotten the "And" in the title. . . . But the "And" is important. It lets us know how cunning the interrogator is, how uncasual his casual-seeming enquiry. . . .*

I feel like an interrogator myself. "When did you last see your father?" I want to warn people: don't underestimate filial grief, don't think because you no longer live with your parents, have had a difficult relationship with them, are grown up and perhaps a parent yourself, don't think that will make it any easier when they die.

Blake Morrison, *And When Did You Last See Your Father?*

Seven years ago, Joan was the hospice nurse for my father, who was dying of brain cancer. She was his favorite among the nurses who would come to care for him. She certainly was the only person whom he would allow to bathe him. Joan, sensing his odd combination of modesty and pride, visited more frequently than necessary, often wearing swimsuits under her clothing so that she could shower with him.

With amazement, I watched her easy tenderness toward this man whose projected reserve had kept even his own children at arm's length. She would actually cuddle with him, *tease him!* My fearsome father, shamefacedly chortling and ducking his pleasure-reddened face! He noticeably brightened at her approach, enlarged upon his feelings in words he had never used with us, expressed anxieties his children would never have suspected.

Emboldened by Joan's success, I decided on a plan of action. Several times, like a cat stalking skittish prey, I approached and feinted, relaxing into a posture of languid indifference if his eye happened toward me. Finally, tensing with my practiced words, I appeared behind him as he stood, doddering, in his study.

He turned around so rapidly that we were suddenly eye to eye, uncomfortably close.

"Daddy," I said, "I love you."

He appeared to recoil slightly and looked confused, then a sweet expression of indulgence suffused his face. He reached out and tenderly patted me on the shoulder.

"There, there, girl," he said.

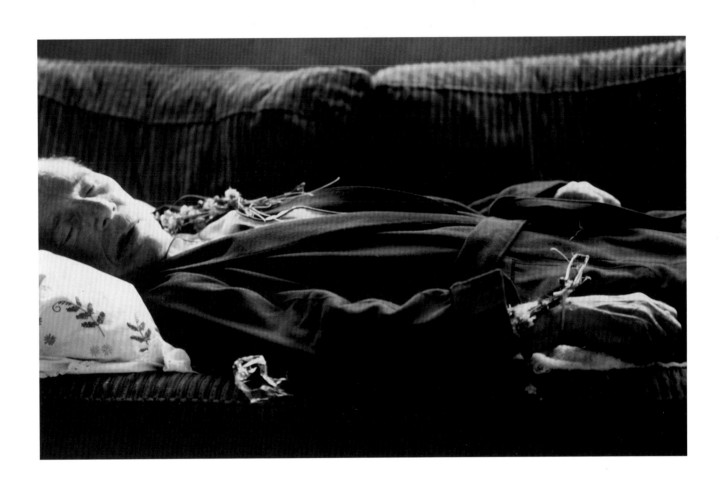

Like so many others, this patient seems to shed an overcoat of worry when Joan and I appear at her back door. Her concerns are myriad: her dying sister's constipation, the telephone arguments with the insurance company, and the unnatural angle of the fake bird wired to the bird feeder outside the sickroom's window. As is so often the case, she is untroubled by the presence of a stranger and, it turns out, I am not such a stranger after all.

"Good Lord, I'd know you *anywhere,*" she exclaims before Joan can finish her introduction. The Hepburn-cheekboned sister rises up from the bed and concurs: "Law, she looks just like her mother." Featherlike, she subsides back into the covers. Her bright bird-eyes follow our motions. Occasionally she corrects her sister, a habit that seems lifelong. She does so with adamantine resolve during an anecdote about my father, who was their family doctor for a disputed number of years.

Joan and I have noticed an unusual willingness to include me in the medical talk at these homes. I have been invited to discuss the efficacy of dosages, share in the lavage of bedsores, and palpate vaginal tumors the size of breadfruit. Here, the virtues of mineral oil over an enema are discussed, and I nod earnestly at the conclusions. Because our hospice program is community-run and family-oriented, when we gather around the patient there is an inclusive familiarity.

But there have been many of these sickbed gatherings at which I've sensed the ghost of my father, and my mirror-image mother. Both are recalled with affection and with nostalgia for the days of victory gardens and house calls. When they speak of my father, it is with a familiar reverence that is peculiar to those who have known a doctor as both an intimate home-care deliverer and as a demigod.

Letting myself out the back door and into the trig little farmyard, its pollarded trees rigid against the gray winter light, I remember my father's horror of pollarding. Then, reproaching myself, I remember his great ability to keep his thoughts to himself. I straighten and rewrap the wires holding the bird on its plastic dowel.

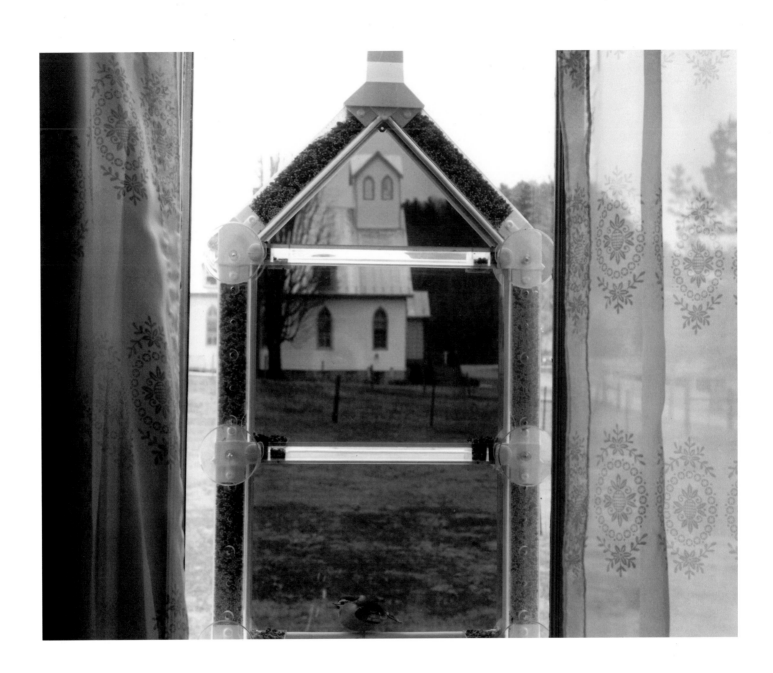

Joan is Jewish and I am a liberal, but our new patient couldn't tell that from looking at us — or if he could, it didn't stop him from offering up opinions that would offend both of us. The recent bombing in Oklahoma was the springboard for a hate-filled polemic about the government's interference in everything (although he failed to acknowledge that federal mining regulations had protected coal miners like himself, or that he and his family have depended on Medicare and welfare).

During this harangue I watch Joan, whose smile hardly dims. The wattage goes down somewhat at the mention of the rich New Jersey Jews who are buying up the countryside, and neither Joan nor I mention that she is from New Jersey. His xenophobic antennae extended, he senses an intruder and accuses me of being a Yankee. The next thing I know, I am testily asserting my Southern roots. This man got to me.

But not to Joan. She ruffles his greasy hair, teases up his shirt to have a listen to his ticker, and massages his gimped-up leg. While she is caring for him, he offers another cautionary tale, this time about niggers. Play-acting the credulous children's parts, as well as proudly reprising his own, he recounts key moments of intimidation and misinformation in the upbringing of his eleven children which appear to have turned all of them into racists.

Meanwhile, Joan smoothes his bed covers and tenderly palpates his back. She inquires after the family, takes the wife's blood pressure, and calls Virginia Power about an overdue bill. Her concern for this man's personal life is not feigned, and her tenderness is unforced. When we leave the house, I am in a rage. Joan benignly waves out her window at his eager face as we drive away.

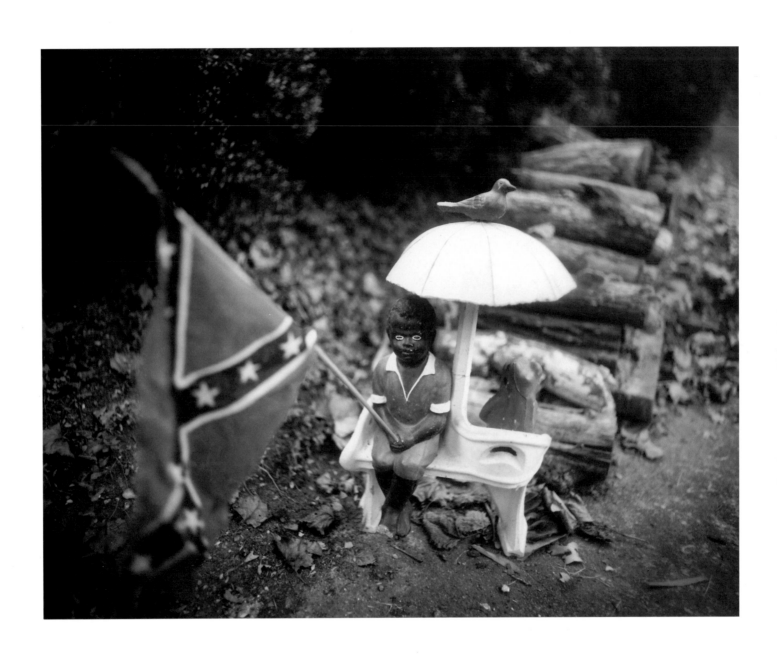

The idea of death, the fear of it, haunts the human animal like nothing else. Heroism is first and foremost a reflex of the terror of death. We admire most the courage to face death . . . it moves us deeply in our hearts because we have doubts about how brave we ourselves would be. When we see a man bravely facing his own extinction we rehearse the greatest victory we can imagine . . . the hero has been the center of human honor and acclaim since probably the beginning of specifically human evolution.

Ernest Becker, *The Denial of Death*

Cancer followed three years of bad luck: a near-fatal car wreck, two prostate operations, and a heart attack. He had emerged from it all as stringy and tough as the jerky he always kept tucked in his shirt pocket. He was a mountain man, born so far up the holler that his first exposure to flat land was at twelve, by which time he had acquired about all the education he would get. He had done so by reading the only two books in his house: the Bible and *Little Black Sambo*. Since he remained unnamed well into his youth, he ended up taking his legal name from the latter.

He was a bear hunter. In his lifetime he had tracked and killed uncounted bears, many of them more than three times his own weight. People attributed his legendary ability to his American Indian blood. Like his counterpart in literature, Faulkner's Sam Fathers, he had been seen to take on a full-grown bear and bring it down with just a knife.

The week before he died, his daughter's full-term baby was born dead. Mindless of, or perhaps because of, the grief in the house, he announced that he was going out to get one last, long-elusive bear. All attempts to discourage him failed, and he followed his eager dogs into the mountains.

He was much weakened, and his tracking was slow and labored. This allowed several hunting friends to secretly shepherd the bear in his direction. Ignorant to the last of the conspiracy, he triumphantly treed and shot his last bear. Both he and the bear were carried home, and he fell into a coma within hours.

On the paper bearing the inked impressions of her dead baby's feet, his daughter wrote a note. It read:

> *Daddy, here's his feet prints. If anyone can track him down in heaven, you can.*

She folded it into a tiny square, and as she saw her father leaving this world, she poked it deep into his pajama pocket.

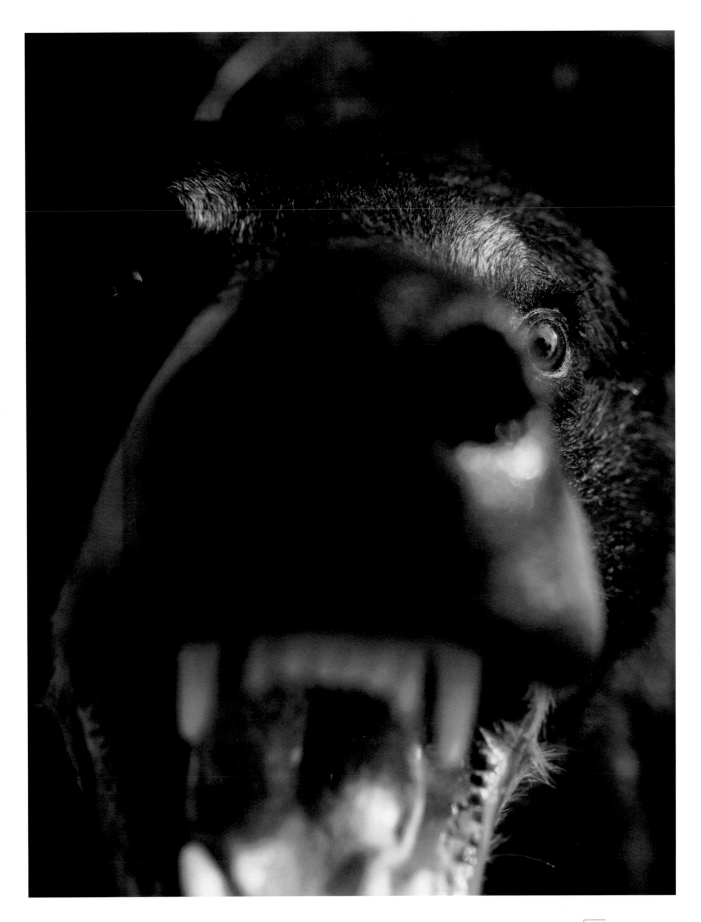

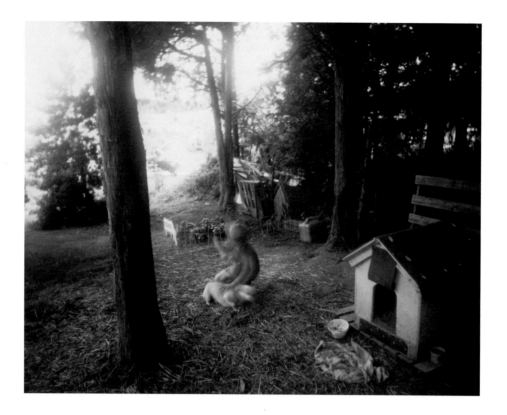

Joan said this patient had been the envy of frazzled householders like the two of us. I reflect on this as I labor up the driveway where she waits for me, my camera bellows drooping off the track like a doleful elephant's trunk and my uncapped lenses grinding together in the chaos of my camera bag. As I toss them in her van, I'm comforted by its familiar clutter: hospice supplies and kid stuff, seats stuck with Sugar Daddies. Joan and I driving down the road look like crazed harridans, our hair tangled, children's school reports fluttering at our feet like autumn leaves.

Not this guy: before he became ill, his life epitomized order. Taped to the inside of every drawer was a list of each object within, supplemented by a grid outlining its exact location. The newer items were placed farther back in the drawer, so that the older ones could enjoy their full utility. He planned his meals a month in advance and prepared the week's meals on Saturday. If well-meaning neighbors brought food to him, he anxiously attempted to divide the offering into seven equal portions.

As he became unable to maintain the structure of his life, he was moved to the home of a professional caregiver. Her house sits on a hummock overlooking the back of a truck stop. The view from the dying man's window is a sea of battered truck bodies, parts strewn like the aftermath of a tornado, trees cut and left where they fell, electrical wires crisscrossing the sky, and plastic bags fluttering like errant banners from the riot of multiflora rose.

We find him agitated and fretful. Looking out of his window, we see a small dog being systematically tortured by neighborhood kids. One of them is holding it down while the other tries to pound a stake down its throat. Sighing, Joan turns away and produces her checkbook.

She asks the old man for help organizing the entries that appear to be written in some form of Sanskrit. His face brightens; he eagerly sets to work. I go outside and tell the boys to pat the dog. When I return to the room, I can see that they are now merely whacking at it, while the patient and Joan bow their heads over his last, greatly reduced sphere of control.

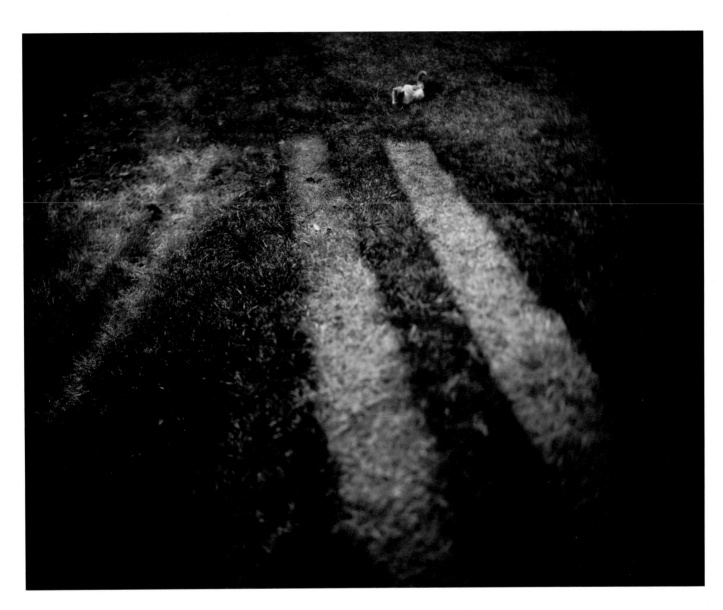

At the count of three, Joan and her assistant hoist the dying man into a wheelchair and roll him from the dark bedroom to a window. With obvious emotion he watches his cat gaily cavorting on the striped stage of etiolated winter lawn. Glancing out, Joan and I remark that it is as if the cat is performing a ballet for him. Taking a longer look, we realize that the patient has been watching the cat torment a small garter snake to death.

Whenever the dullness of the profane was left behind, whenever life grew more intense in whatever way through honor or death . . . marriage or prayer . . . purification or mourning, anything and everything that stirred a person and demanded a meaning, the Greeks would celebrate with fluttering strips of wool, white, for the most part, which they tied around their heads or arms or to a branch. . . . To the Greek eye it was those light fluttering strips of wool that generated meaning, gave it its boundaries, celebrated it. Everything that took place in the soft frame of those woolen strips was different and separate from the rest. What was it those . . . strips, those tassels represented? An excess, a flowing wake that attached itself to a being or thing. And, at the same time, a tether that bound that being or thing.

Isidore of Seville could still write, "Vittae dictae sunt, quod vinciant," "The ties are so called because they bind." But what was this bond? It was the momentary surfacing of a link in that invisible net which enfolds the world, which descends from heaven to earth, binding the two together and swaying in the breeze. . . . [E]very time someone achieves or is subjected to . . . something that uplifts him and generates intensity and meaning, then the ties come out.

All these strips, these vain winged tassels, were nerves of the nexus rerum, the connection of everything with everything else, which alone gives meaning to life. . . . We feel them blowing about us the minute something happens to dispel our apathy, and we become aware of being carried along on a stream that flows toward something unknown. And just sometimes, but very rarely, those ties twist and turn and weave around us, until one loose end becomes knotted to another. Then, very softly, they encompass us, they form a circle, which is the crown, perfection.

Roberto Calasso, *The Marriage of Cadmus and Harmony*

These white strips of cloth could be seen blowing in the breeze long before we saw the woman waving to us from the doorway of the farmhouse. She had tied them to the tree branches to keep her mother, whose eyesight was failing, from hitting her head. This bench was her mother's favorite seat on the property. After her death, the family gathered beneath the fluttering strips of cloth and, unmindful of the Greeks, Isidore of Seville, or any circle of perfection, they held a brief memorial.

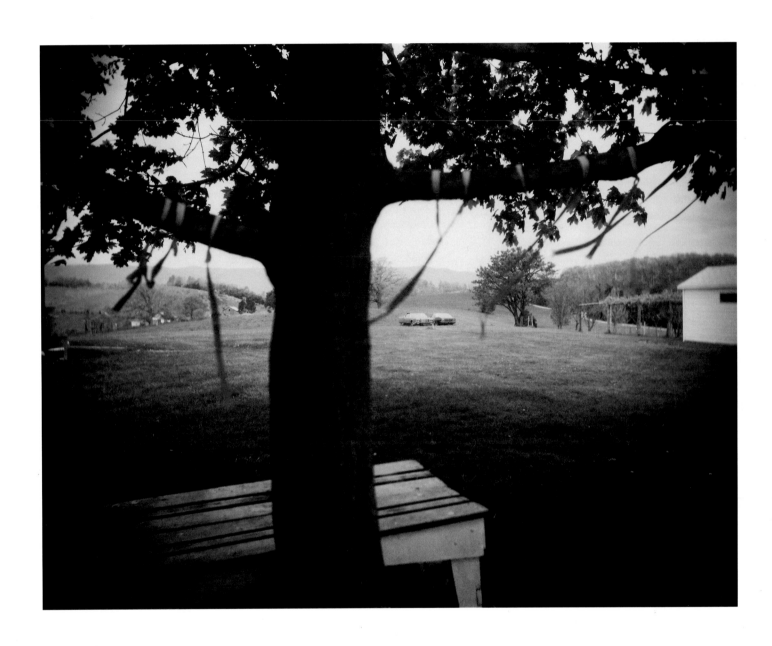

Joan only had this patient for a week before he died. Actually, nobody had had him long, and there wasn't a clue as to where he'd come from. When Joan and I found him he was at an adult care facility, the kind of place where the deinstitutionalized, the impoverished, and the homeless are sent to live out their days and where his, clearly, were numbered.

He gave us the name of a sister who, when contacted, said to fuck off. When he died, Joan held his tiny hand. He was no bigger than we were, and about our age, but life had dished out some bad knocks — starting early we guessed, since he told us he had begun drinking when he was nine.

A week or so after he died, Joan and I were in the director's office at the adult home. She held up a black box that she told us held his ashes. Joan asked her when the services would be. The director's face took on the weary look with which the long-initiated regard the neophytes. She indicated a shelf which was buckling under black boxes identical to the one she held in her arms. "What services?" she asked unnecessarily.

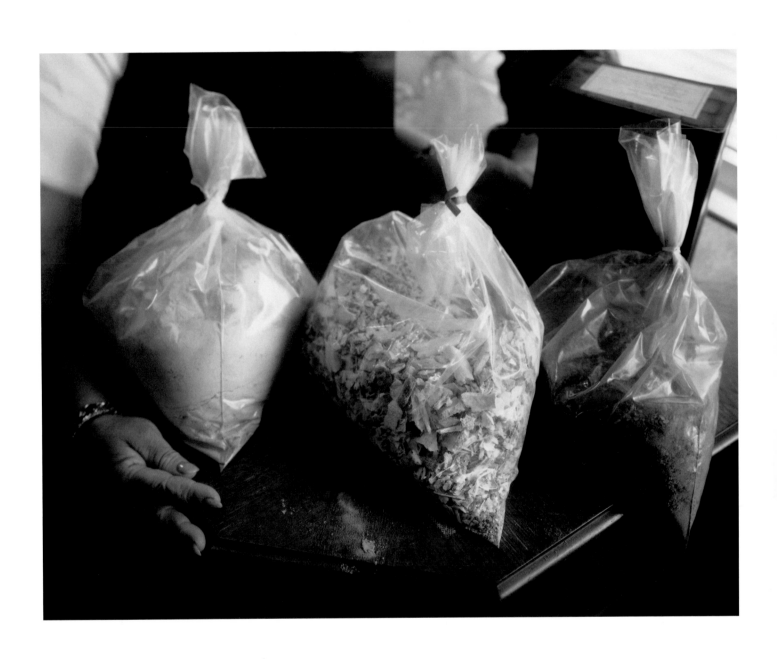

South River runs next to the single-level, simple house of one of Joan's patients who is now in the terminal stage of his illness. There is evidence everywhere of this man's relationship with the river: he has created a swimming hole by damming it up with rock, and he's built pagodas, overlooks, and pavilions on its banks. His crowning achievement, painstakingly pieced together with scraps of wood and strands of wire, is a swinging bridge.

Each time Joan visits, he insists on offering her money, producing a crumpled fifty-dollar bill from a Mason jar by the bed. After a few weeks of this, he apologizes to her for the crude materialism of this gesture and, with the unimpeachable gravity of the moribund, produces a large black plastic key. Puzzled, Joan turns it over and dangles it by a ring from her index finger.

The patient, with a fervid clasp of her wrist, explains to her that this is the key to the river. She must always keep it with her, he cautions, because this key is the only sure way to peace. His solemnity indicates the importance of the gift, and Joan accepts it politely. When she returns to the office she hangs it, with some care, above her desk.

 On our next visit, after a week of rain, the swinging bridge dangles like a broken arm over the river, and Joan's patient lives only a day past its destruction.

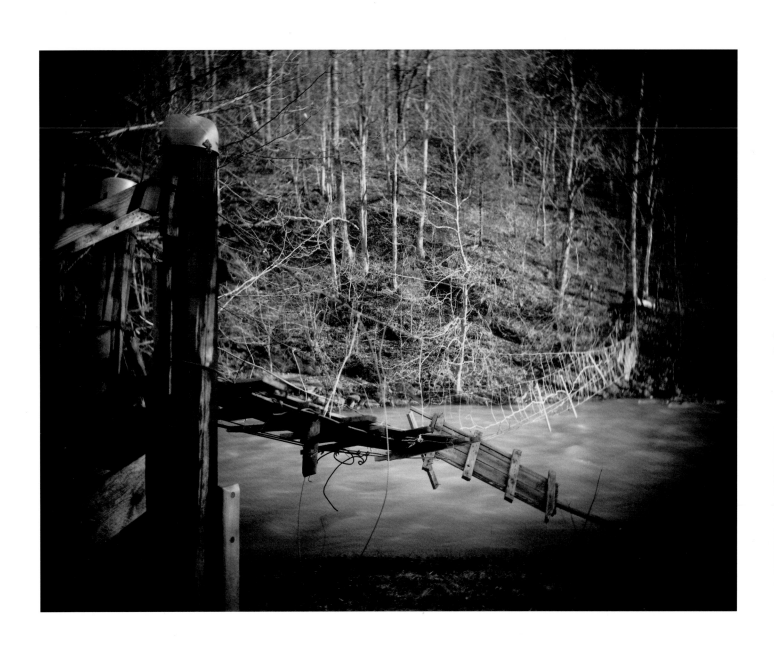

Joan suggested I come with her to see a patient who is dying of cancer of the small intestine. She had lost most of it to surgery and was thin, but claimed to feel fine. Her husband is a large man and seemed especially so next to his delicate wife. Indeed, there was a burly, brutish air about him which, for Joan, was what made his tenderness in looking after his wife so striking. He had even invented what Joan deemed a patentable device for emptying the colostomy.

I went out to see them because I wanted to learn something about the relativity of suffering. I wanted to know if grief is quantifiable, if all deaths are equal in the toll that they take. We spoke about how they contain their fear, sadness, and anger. This is their story, told with obvious anguish.

Five years ago their fifteen-year-old son was beaten to death. The boy was living in town with his sister and her husband. Two days before the boy was killed, the sister's husband broke a finger of his right hand hitting the child. The hand was encased in a hard cast.

The night he was killed, the boy had been caught hitchhiking and brought to the police station. He told the police that he was being beaten and that he was scared to go back to his sister's house. He was so scared that he peed his pants when the police made him go.

He was beaten again that night and died of a ruptured diaphragm. The emergency room nurse reported that his testicles were impossible to locate; she said they had been "shattered."

The sister's husband stood trial and was acquitted. The reasoning laid before the receptive jury was this: since the boy had ingested a possibly lethal dose of a prescription drug, he might have died anyway. He was therefore, in the defense attorney's words, "a fully depreciated victim."

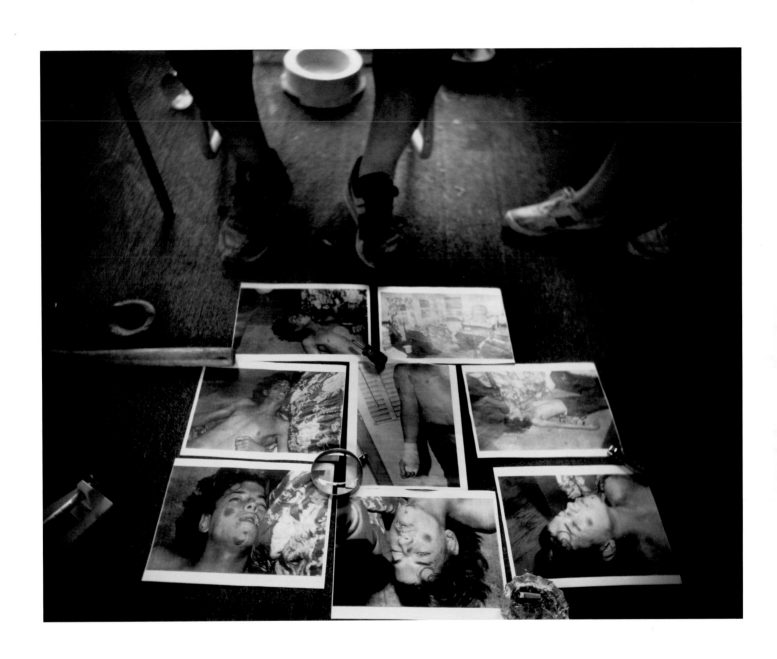

On Valentine's Day Joan took me to visit one of her patients who lived in a house so bleak it looked abandoned. There was a big production at the door. After much knocking, a shriveled, bony arm reached up, pulled the curtain back to check, and opened up an ungenerous slice of doorway.

As soon as we squeezed inside and past the toothless gatekeeper, we could tell Joan's patient was beside himself with impatience. He sat in the overheated, low-ceilinged living room, naked save his underwear. The lower part of his face appeared to be sucked in as if by some internal vortex. At the end of his femur, the knee bones poked through their papery covering of skin. In his excitement they knocked together. When Joan sat on the couch next to him, he reached both hands out and clasped hers. After her initial professional inquiries, his gaze intensified, his grasp tightened, and he shifted around in the classic lover's posture. Joan met his gaze with unfeigned fervor, and with an effort he worked up a lungful and began to sing.

For all the eight stanzas of the love song about the girl in the gingham dress, Joan's eyes never left his. I realized that this was a song that Joan had heard many, many Tuesdays, but I had no idea how many times we were to hear it that particular Valentine's Tuesday. Leaving Joan rapt on the couch, I eventually took my camera into the backyard. I pointed it toward the porch and the frozen underpants hanging from a wire. There, unfocused on the milky ground glass, were two rigid white valentines.

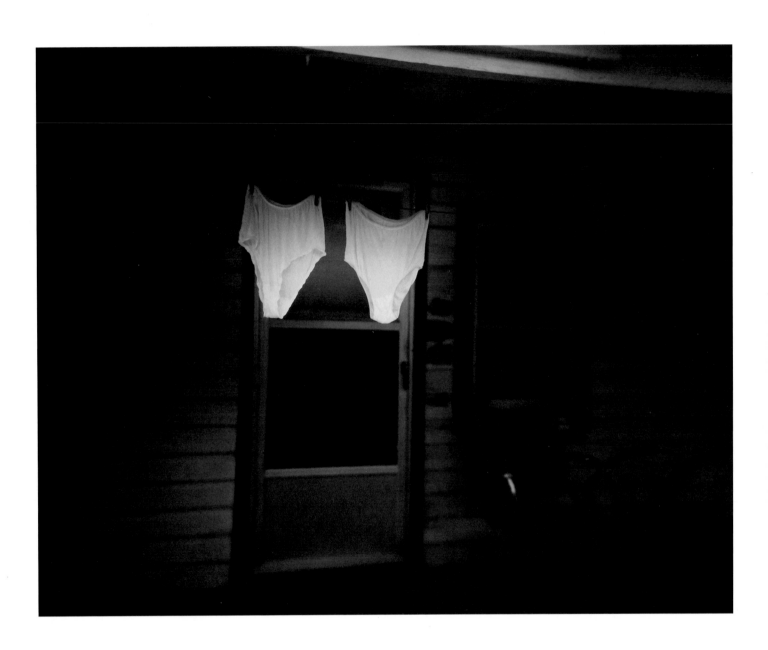

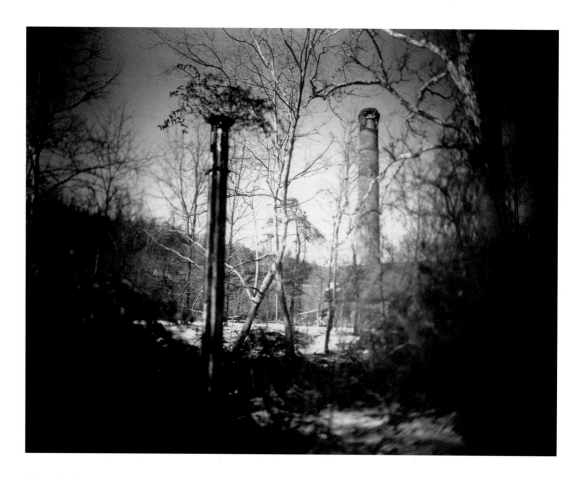

Towards the very end, with a voice that could barely produce a sound, his grandfather told him that he had begun to remember his life. He had been dredging up the days of his Toronto boyhood, reliving events that had taken place as far back as 80 years ago . . . all the trivial, long-forgotten things that now, coming back to him as he lay immobilized in bed, took on the importance of spiritual illuminations. "Lying here gives me a chance to remember," he told A. . . . . Memory was the only thing keeping him alive, and it was as though he wanted to hold off death for as long as possible in order to go on remembering.

Paul Auster, *The Invention of Solitude*

The hospice workers with whom I have spoken tell me that they try to make sure their patients can get a last look at the places they remember.

This was the site of an old furnace from which the patient's father would return nightly, grimy from handling the pig iron. The hospice worker who drove the patient here reports that the sight of the forge brought back memories almost a century old.

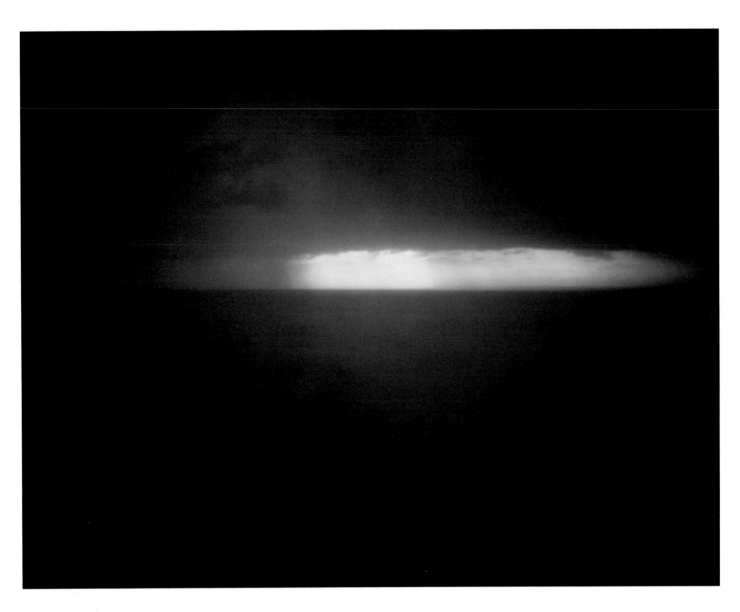

One hospice worker reports driving 250 miles to take a patient to see the ocean one last time.

JACK RADCLIFFE

Philip Brookman: What brought you to work with the people that you did?

Jack Radcliffe: I had mixed feelings when I was asked to participate in this project. I'm always excited about new opportunities, but I wasn't sure how or if this fit into my work. When I began, I wasn't really sure what hospice was. I only knew that it had to do with death. One of my students was a nurse. When I asked her about hospice, she put me in touch with Joy Ufema, founder of York House Hospice in York, Pennsylvania. I sent a letter to Joy and when she invited me to photograph at the hospice, I was extremely apprehensive. However, at this time in my life it was fortuitous. My mother had just died, and my father was dying. I wasn't dealing at all with my loss. Being with Joy and the nurses at York House — seeing their devotion to their patients, both physical and spiritual — helped me to view death as a part of life. It was a cathartic transformation for me, and eventually I was able to grieve for my parents as well as the patients I came to know.

PB: What unique experiences did you have working at York House?

JR: For the first year it was a struggle for me to work there because of the emotional intensity. I'd never before photographed someone whom I didn't relate to in some way. I had always relied on my ability to interact with my subjects. But the first person I photographed at York House, Pete, was blind and deaf. I'm not sure if he was even conscious of my presence. This was a terribly difficult experience. I didn't want to go back. For a while I was filled with dread every time I went to the hospice. But when I saw Joy and the nurses, their kindness and love won me over. It made a big difference that I felt I was a part of the hospice effort, rather than an outsider documenting an event.

PB: What did you set out to accomplish and how did you develop it?

JR: I really didn't understand hospice when I began. As I learned about it, my experience became very personal since my parents hadn't been in hospice care. I realized how different their experience was. So I didn't want to make just another series of pictures of sick people. I wanted to show these patients as people with names, personalities, and identities. For example, Sheila was a lovely woman who had a difficult life. In her last months she made it her mission to talk to people about AIDS. She wanted to know exactly how my pictures would be used before giving permission to photograph. "Will they teach people about AIDS?" she asked. When she was satisfied, I thought I'd be allowed to photograph right away. "Come back next week," she said. "I'll have my hair done." I wanted to show this side of her.

PB: How is this project different from your previous work?

JR: In my previous work I was always striving for intimacy. In a way, this project forced me to achieve a new level of intimacy. At York House I photographed over and over in the same three rooms. I wanted to reveal the relationship of my subjects to their environment. Soon I had to find new visual solutions to this problem. I changed my perspective and moved in closer to the patients. This realization, in turn, has transformed my photography.

PB: What did you hope to reveal in your photographs?

JR: Photographs of suffering people are commonplace. Some photographers stay at a safe distance or romanticize their subjects. Others either protect or assault the viewer. I didn't want my pictures to have either effect. I wanted them to be genuine. I tried to be confrontational yet empathetic, to share and record real moments. I wanted to share not only my experiences but the patients' experiences as well.

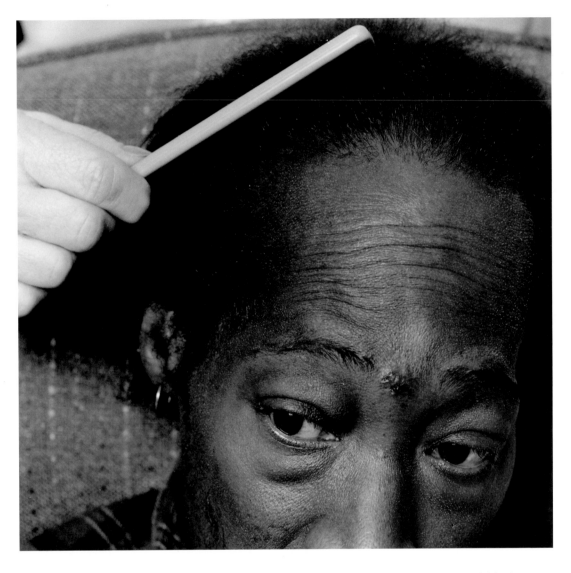

Gill, February 24, 1995

Joy tells us that Gill's wife, Jackie, left him because of his drug use and refused to take him back as long as he was using, but she returned to help him die.

Barbara Ellen Wood

Captions are excerpted from a journal by Barbara Ellen Wood and interviews with Jack Radcliffe, Joy Ufema, and Carolyn Copenheaver.

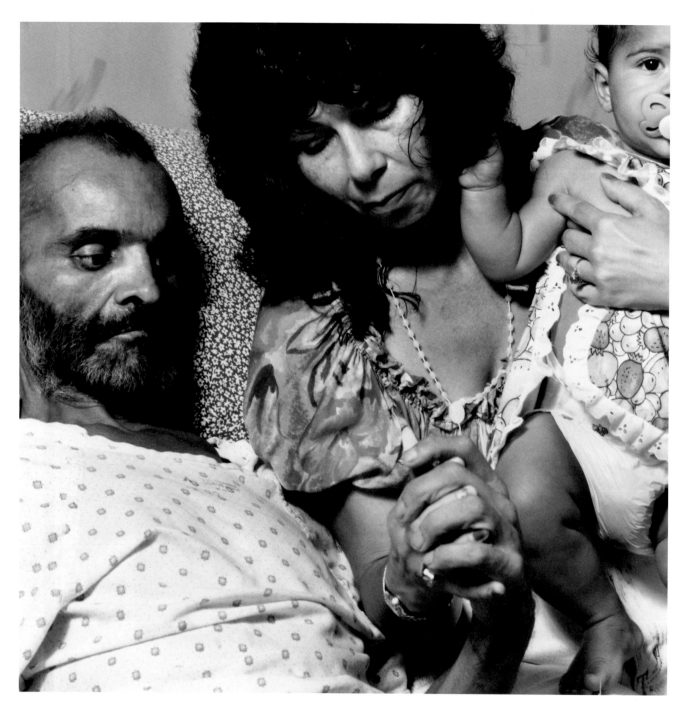

Honky with Heidi and Rikki
August 19, 1994

"Honky's good to me," Rikki says. "He never hits me."

Jack Radcliffe

Jimmy with Jody and Jimiel
March 3, 1995

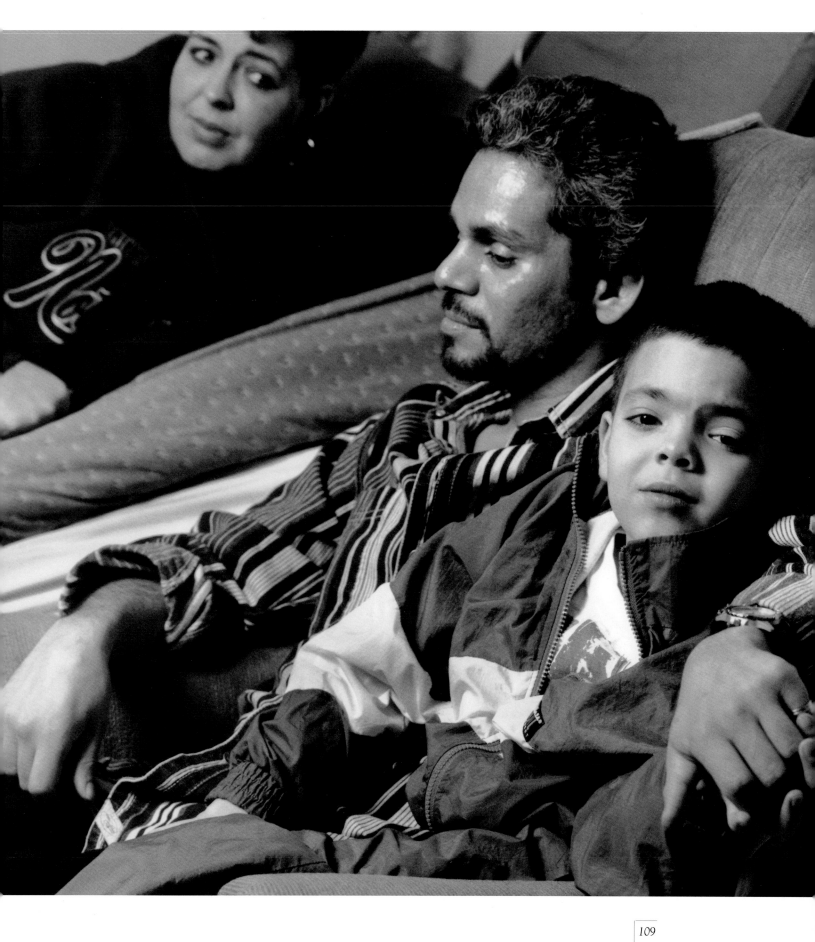

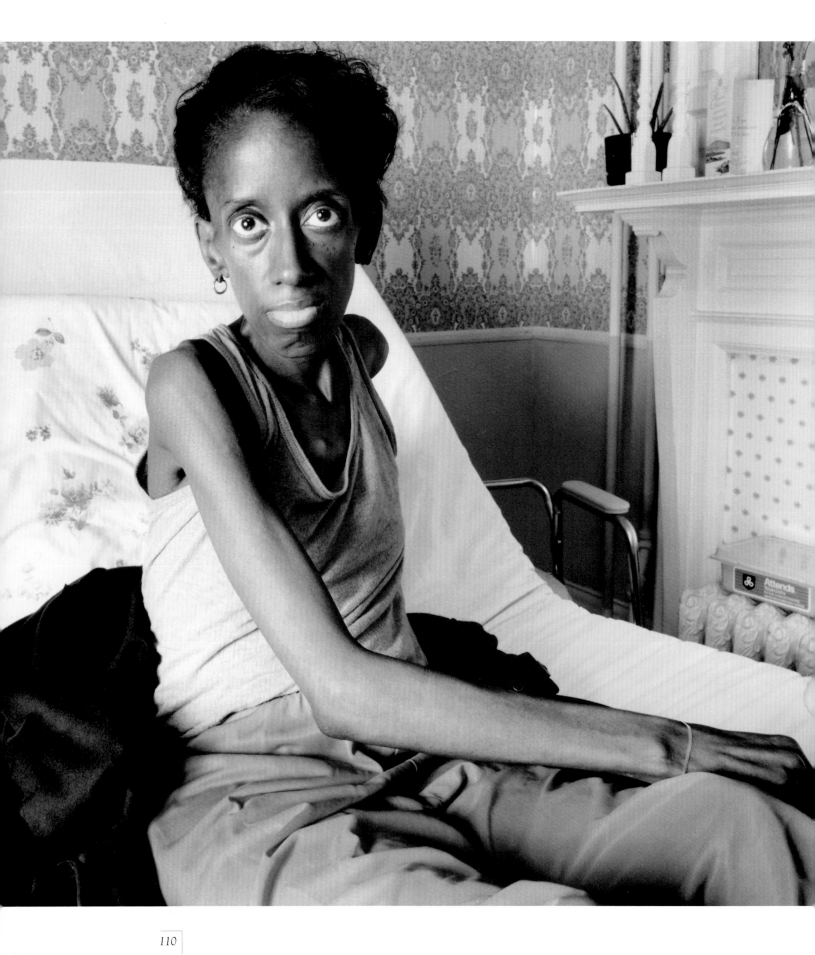

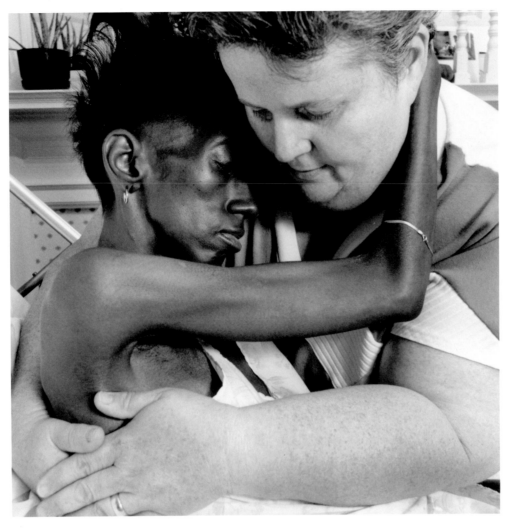

Sheila and Georgia
July 14, 1992

Sheila is not a passive subject in these pictures. She directs and stages scenes that, for her, describe the daily ordeal of having AIDS.

Barbara Ellen Wood

Sheila, July 3, 1992

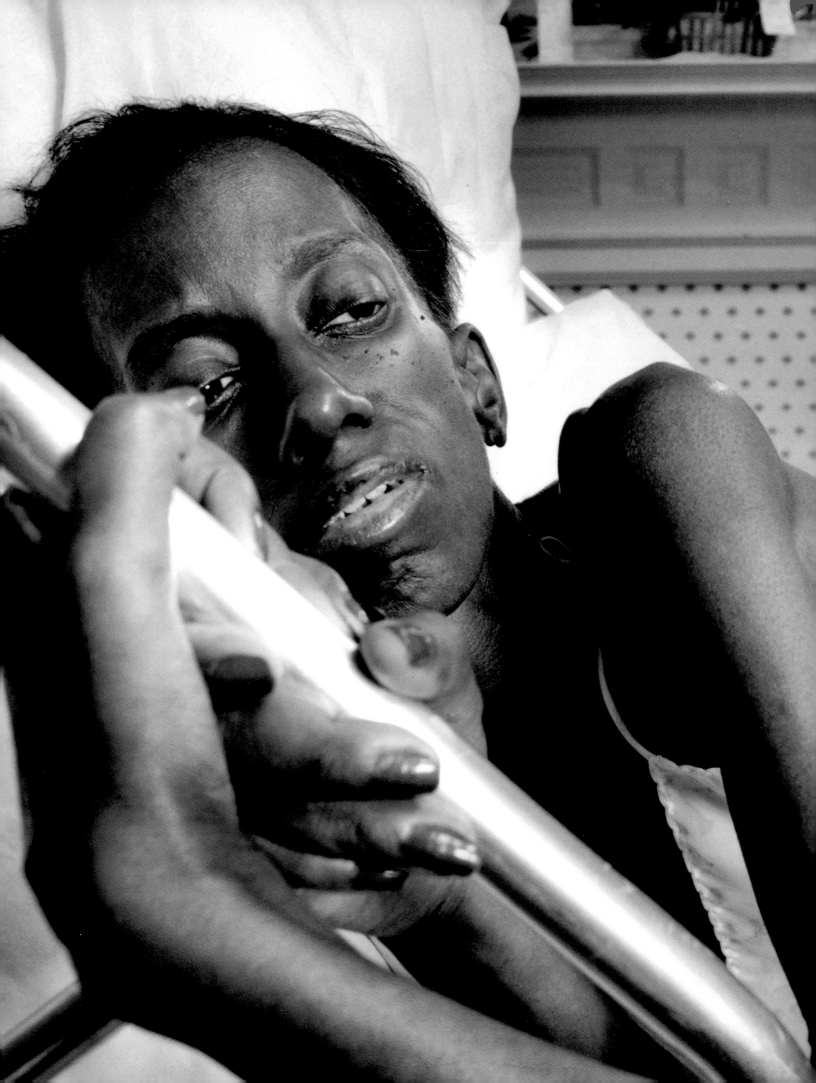

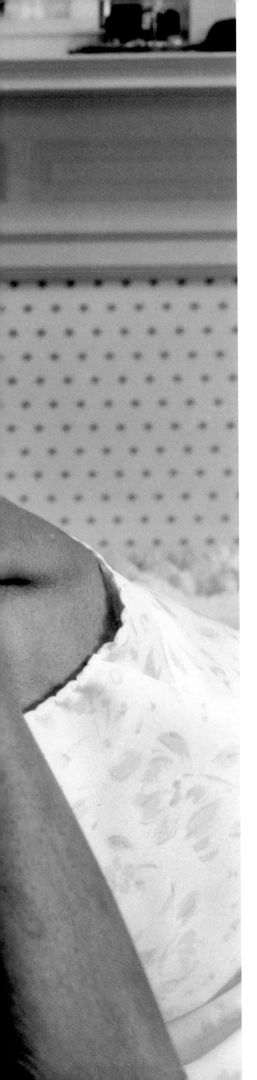

Sheila, July 14, 1992

Sheila has shrunk noticeably in the ten days since we last saw her. She has also grown more visibly ill. I could not imagine where she was going to find the strength to endure the photo session.

Barbara Ellen Wood

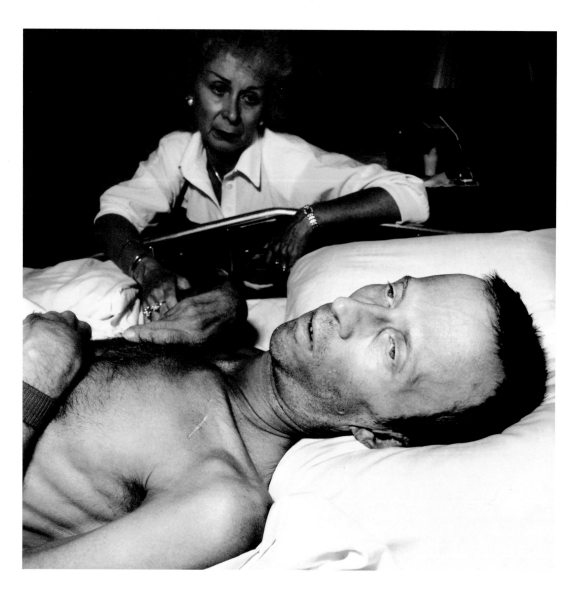

Pete and a Friend
June 14, 1992

Pete's wife, Nancy, recalls that Pete's last words to her before he lapsed into a coma were, "Good-bye, Toots."

Barbara Ellen Wood

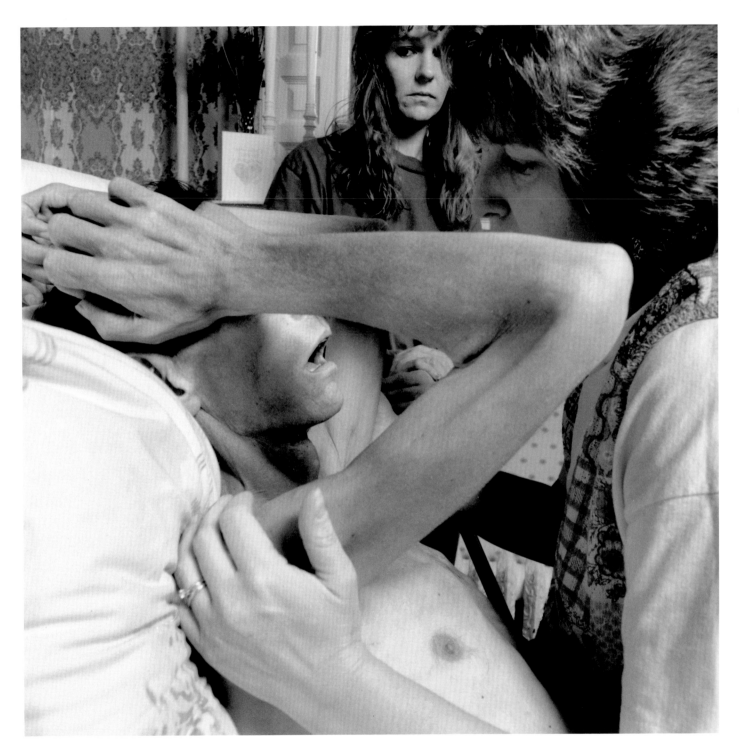

As I photographed Barnie, I felt like such an intruder.
I had to repeat to myself, "These people want me to
document this."

Jack Radcliffe

Barnie with Patricia and Lisa
November 4, 1994

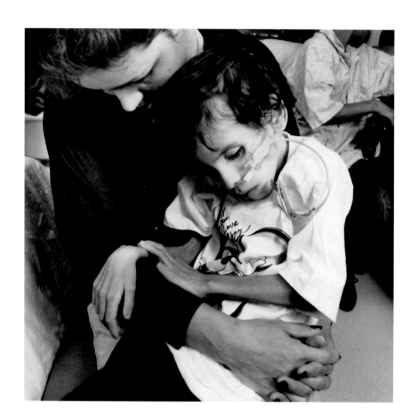

His sixth birthday was coming up and he told me he
was not going to die on his birthday because that
would make his mother sad. When we started with
his death work, we reminded him that at any time he
wanted to lift off, he could be a bright red balloon —
lift off when he was ready — because his body was
very broken, but the Boo Boo in him could fly and
ride horses in the sky, just soar. And he grasped
that. He died two days after his birthday.

Joy Ufema

Boo Boo with His Mother, Luz
April 2, 1993

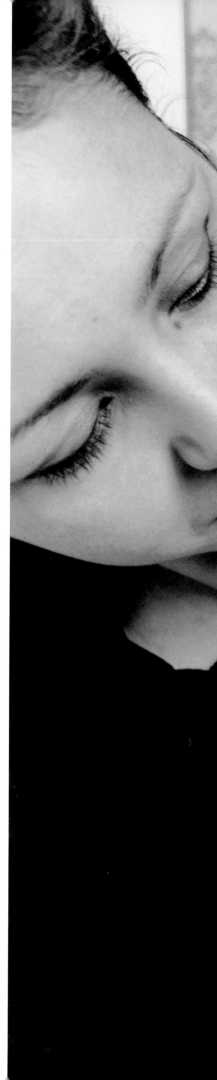

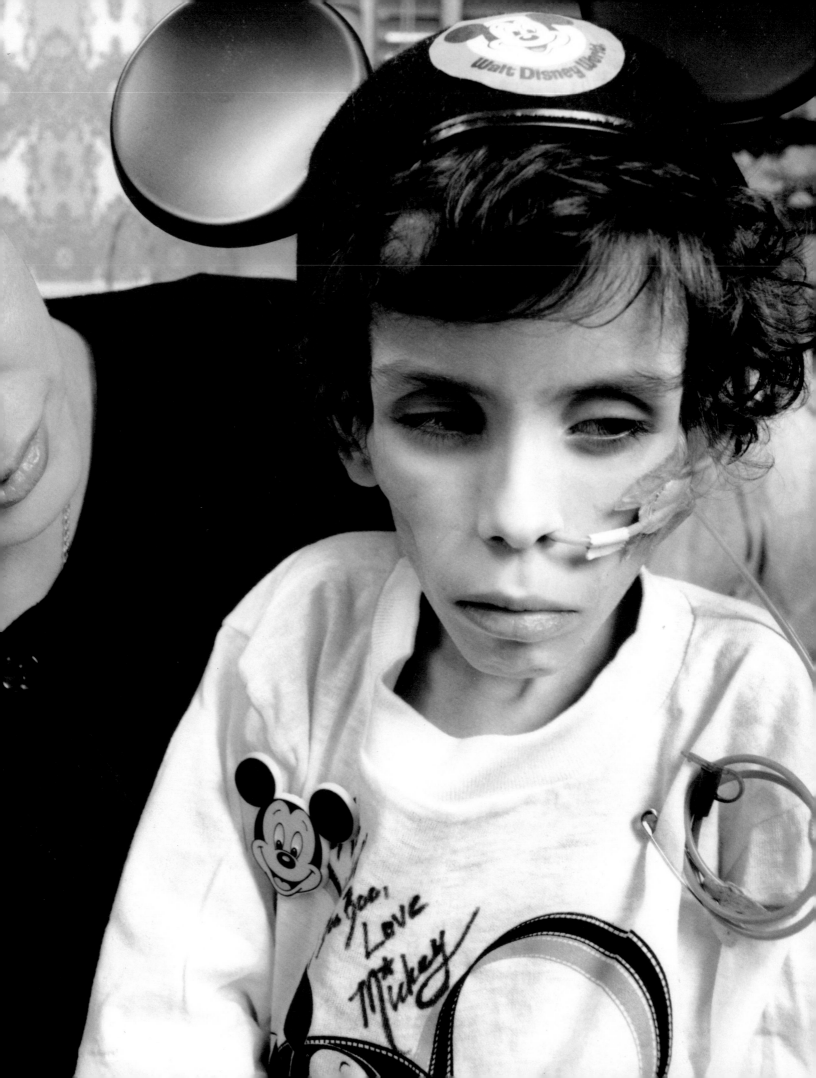

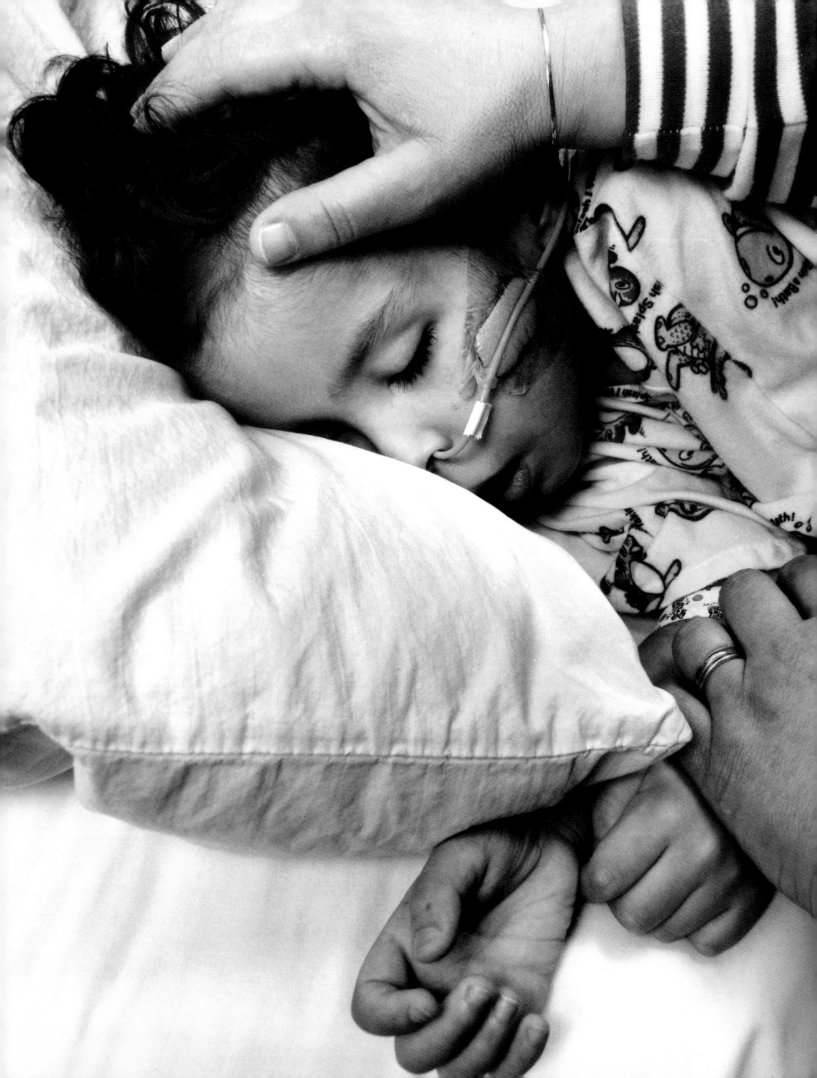

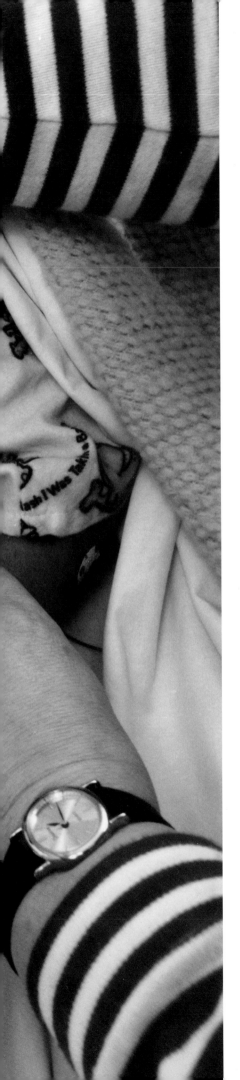

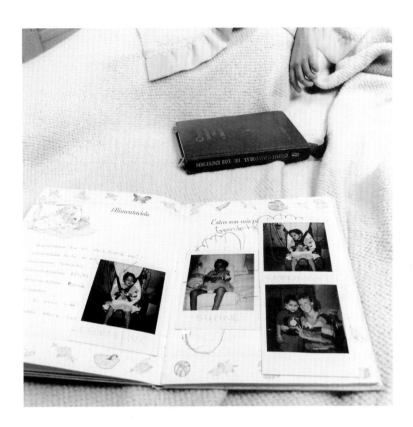

Boo Boo was born April 10, 1987. He has been loved and treasured, and his life recorded diligently in his baby book, which is with him in his room at the hospice.

Boo Boo's siblings have already lost their father, are about to lose an aunt, and now are losing their baby brother as well as their mother — also dying from AIDS.

Barbara Ellen Wood

Boo Boo, March 26, 1993

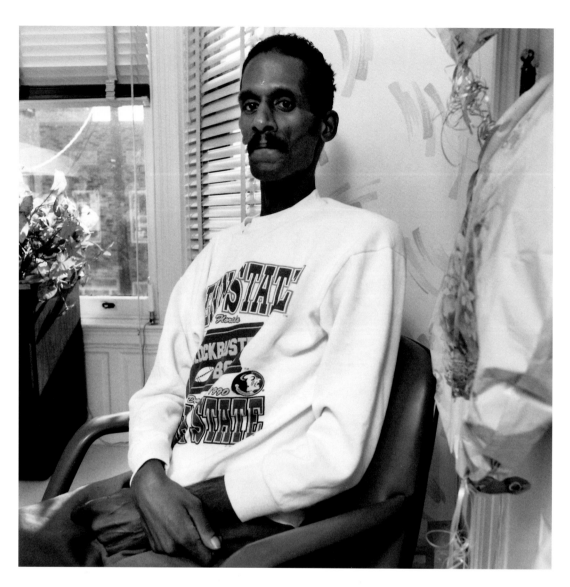

Richard
August 21, 1992

Richard's wife, Maggie, has still not arrived. . . . Richard is clearly upset that she has not appeared as planned. His cough has grown worse and consumes his energy with each spasm. He is not as talkative as usual, which may be due to Maggie's absence or his diminished strength, or both.

Barbara Ellen Wood

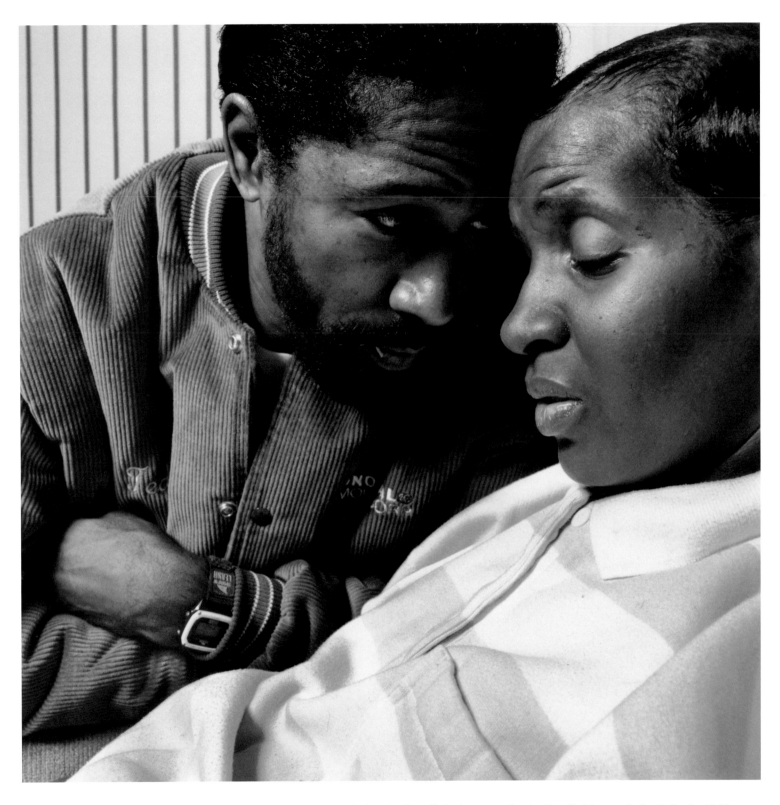

Jack asks Cory if she has seen her brother Teddy.
She angrily yells, "Don't mention that name to me."
Just then Teddy enters. He seems to have a way
with her, because she softens as he touches her.

Barbara Ellen Wood

*Richard's Brother Teddy
and Sister Cory*
December 18, 1992

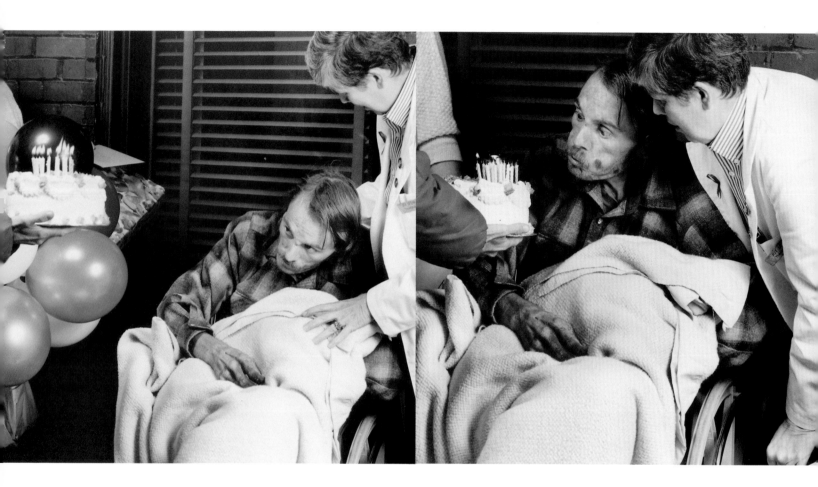

Randy's 33rd Birthday
October 15, 1993

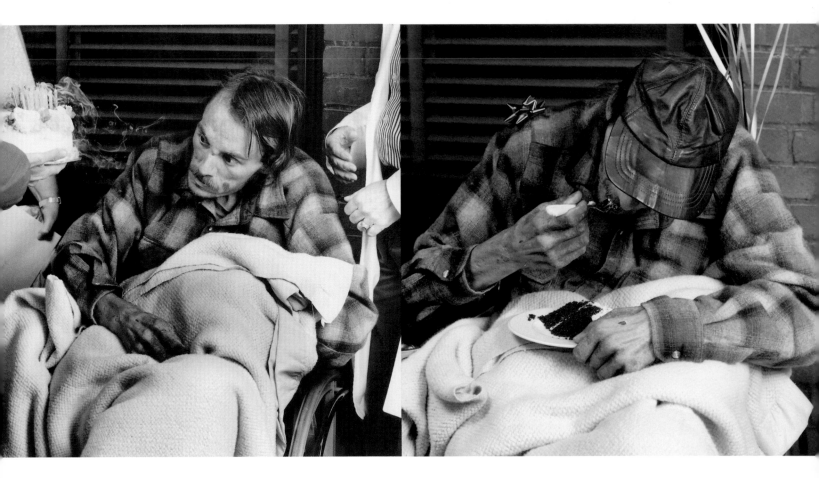

Carolyn Copenheaver, a hospice nurse, told me a little of Randy's story. He left home at twenty after his mother was killed in an auto accident. He'd been on the streets since that time . . . although there was a short time when he had a wife and son in Ohio. Randy's sisters and brothers met their nephew for the first time at York House Hospice.

I am surprised at how much Randy seems to enjoy all the attention: the singing, the candles, and especially the gifts. The staff brought things they knew he would appreciate, mostly warm clothes — coat, hat, long underwear — since he refuses to come indoors except to eat or sleep.

Barbara Ellen Wood

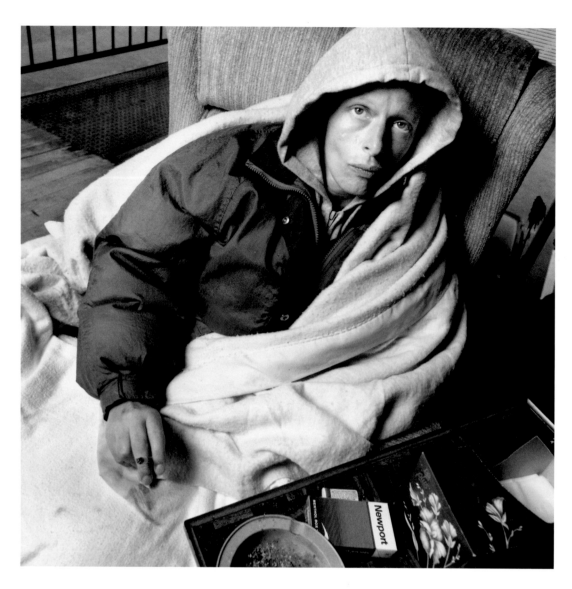

Mary
December 16, 1994

Mary would tell us about her son, whom she left with her husband when he was four years old. Joy called him and explained the situation, and the next day we heard the doorbell and when I answered the door there was a young man. He came in and said he was Mary's son, Billy. So I took him upstairs — Mary was on the porch smoking, even though it was really cold out. And I said, "Mary, look who's here." She looked past me and saw him and said, "I don't know who that is." And I said, "Mary, this is your son, Billy." Mary didn't have any tears to cry because her tear ducts had dried up, but it was sort of a sob that came out of her. He brought her a dozen roses that day. We put the roses in water and put them right beside her bed and nursed them along. I think they lasted about a week and a half. She was just so happy with those roses and that she had found her son again.

Carolyn Copenheaver

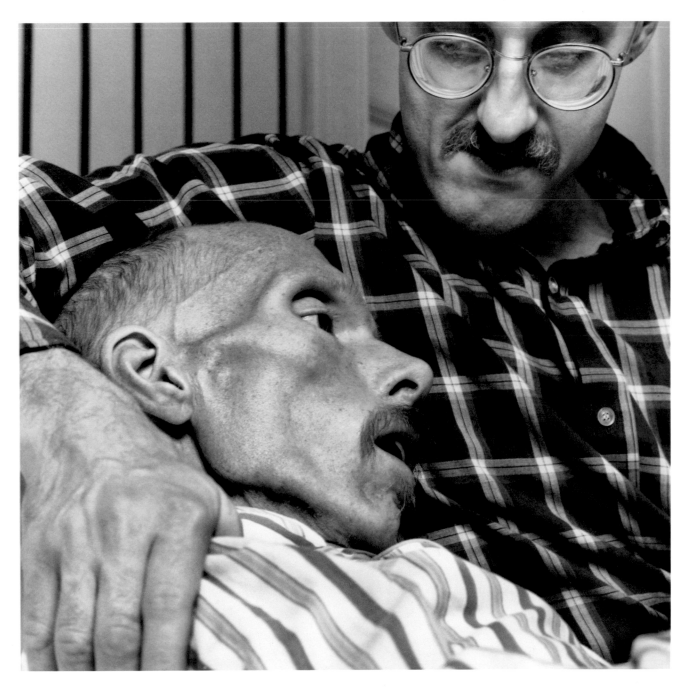

When we enter Larry's room, his friend Frank is feeding him. They agree to be photographed and, though most of our time with them is spent in silence, there is an unspoken communication between them that our intrusion doesn't interrupt.

Barbara Ellen Wood

Larry and Frank
November 4, 1994

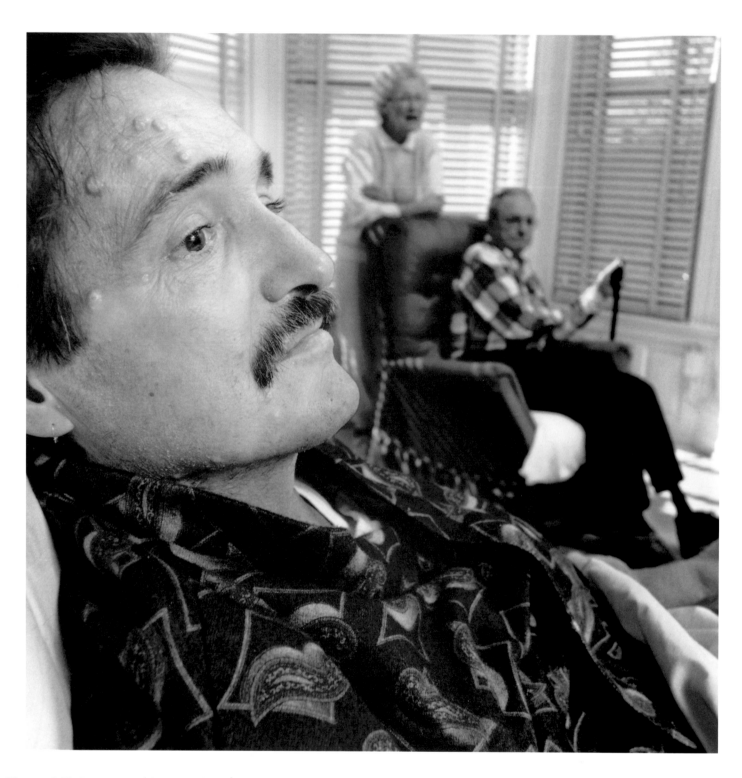

Wayne with His Parents,
Pearl and Charlie
February 26, 1993

It is not as if Pearl won't let Wayne speak, but I have the feeling that she believes that if she keeps talking, her words will be like a blanket that covers him and keeps him safe.

Barbara Ellen Wood

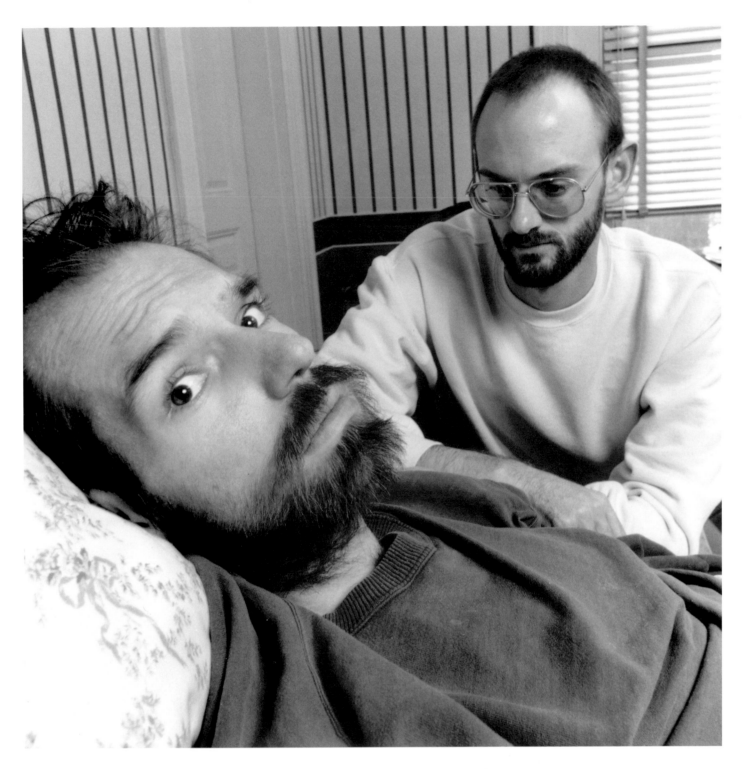

When I return to Rogen's room to say good-bye, I tell him that I won't shake his hand this time because I realize how much it hurts him. He takes my hand, strokes it, while he tells me that it is better to feel a little pain than to miss receiving any affection.

Barbara Ellen Wood

Rogen and Dave
November 13, 1992

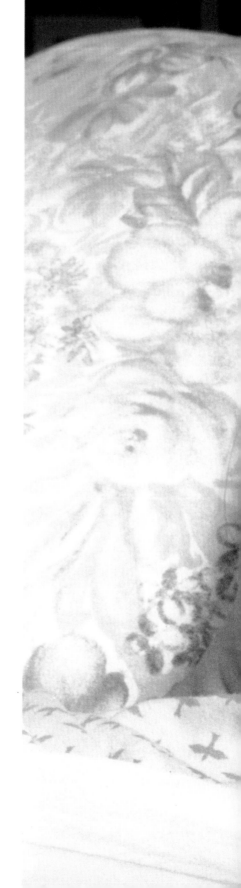

We arrive at 2:30 to photograph Judy, and learn that she died a couple of hours earlier. Her sister, Dottie, says she would like Jack to do a portrait, since it had been Judy's wish. A little while later, Joy and Ginny, a hospice nurse, come downstairs looking for scissors and an envelope so they can cut a lock of Judy's hair and give it to her friend Bill.

Barbara Ellen Wood

Judy, October 25, 1992

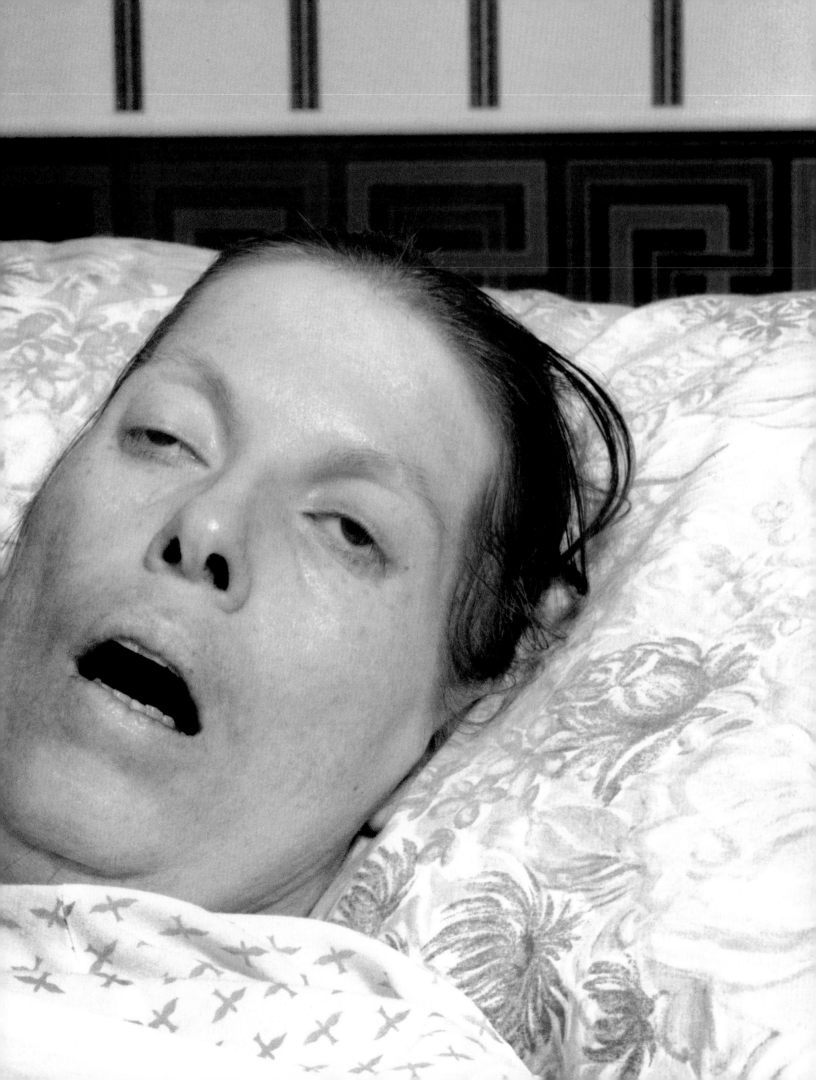

KATHY VARGAS

Philip Brookman: Describe your project.

Kathy Vargas: If one is remembered, then one lives on. I worked with the complementary concepts of life, death, and memory, and the idea of remembrance as eternity. My project is about the lives of a few people who died and about the essence of their memories. I created shrines from these memories. It is also about the "memory-carriers," who are usually the primary caregivers or health-care professionals who treat these people and who continue to remember them. I didn't specifically go looking for my subjects. They found me. People who wanted to talk — to tell the story of hospice and their loved ones — shared their memories with me.

PB: What did you set out to accomplish?

KV: I wanted to remember and celebrate those who were gone, because they were so loved and valued by their families and friends. I also wanted to thank hospice, on behalf of those people, for making a difficult time more bearable and meaningful.

PB: What methods did you employ in this project and how is it different from your previous work?

KV: This project became more like my other work than I thought it would. I have usually made art with and about people I know. But if a stranger is telling you about a person they've loved very deeply, who is now gone, whatever distance there was closes really fast. When you are recording people's most precious memories, when they give you the essence of those who have filled their lives with joy, it's impossible not to put yourself right there with them. The concept of making shrines for people comes from my Chicano background, from my grandmother. I learned to construct altars, offer *milagros,* or enshrine that which is precious, as a way of mediating between the earthbound forces I can control and the "powers that be," such as God, or fate, which I don't control and which determine things like death. The shrines in my hospice work are humanistic, "secular" shrines. They enshrine the memory of the deceased. These shrines are my cultural response to the universal reality of death. I relate shrines to photographs, with their silver, their references to preserving that which is precious to us, and the ability to encode a memory. I've always been in awe of the ability of photographs to preserve a specific time, to be a physical memory. Photography is a mediation between that moment we can control, when an image is made, and those beyond our control, in which the image will continue its life without us.

PB: What unique experiences did you have?

KV: I knew that hospices were very special spaces, but I didn't know why and I was curious. There was a calm and a kindness that I could never fathom. Now I understand. There's an incredible amount of love going out to the person leaving and to the family feeling this loss. One can try to portray that love, but the actuality is infinitely more intense. It's not "normal" to face death calmly and with dignity. Our society generally doesn't discuss death calmly or discuss it at all. To experience the relative calm of those in the process of departing, the sanity of the family members saying good-bye, the devotion of hospice workers, and the acceptance of death as something at once special and ordinary was unique for me. Experiencing hospice is like being given the "grace" to live and experience the whole of life, even as it is ending.

PB: Is it possible to record the passing of life?

KV: I'm less interested in the passing of life than in its persistence. It's easy to see when life has passed. The body becomes useless and the essence of life goes elsewhere. That "elsewhere" is different for everyone, depending on what one believes. But the essence of the life of the beloved always dwells in the memories of those who continue to love and remember. I want to show that persistence of love and memory, along with the role hospice plays in encouraging it. That's what my work is about.

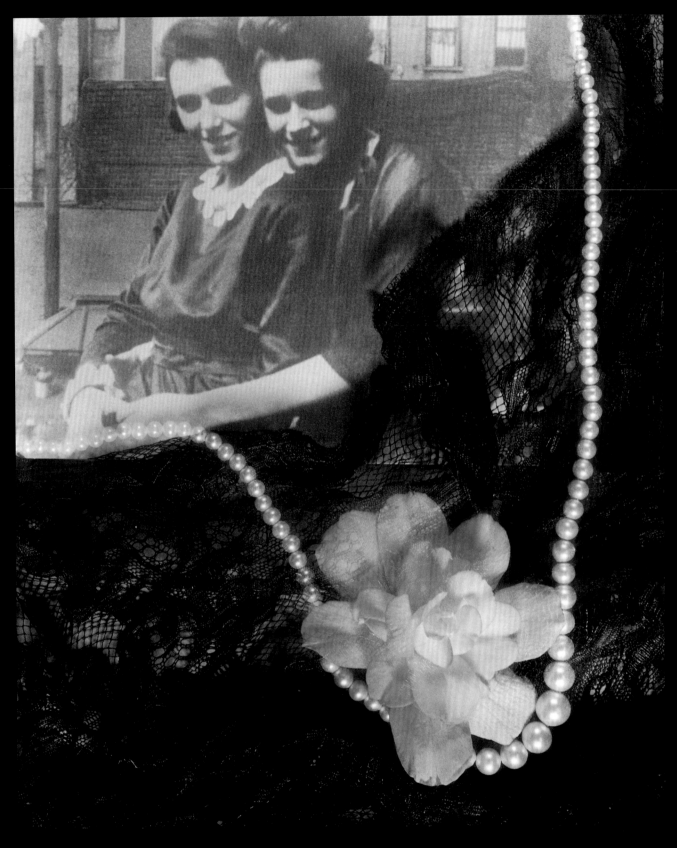

Maria Towne:
Maria with Her Sister Cecelia Grammas, 1994

San Antonio AIDS Foundation, 1994
The San Antonio AIDS Foundation operates a residence that works with the Santa Rosa Hospice. Interview with Patrick Day

Patrick Day: I've been a hospice nurse about six years. I work at the Santa Rosa Hospice and I was "gifted" to the foundation because, at the time, I was one of the only male nurses on the Santa Rosa staff and my supervisor thought AIDS patients would relate better to me, and in fact I think they have. I believe there are very few people I deal with who don't have a feeling of trust.

While working with the foundation, I got a lot more comfortable dealing with AIDS patients. At one point I had left nursing to get away from AIDS. I didn't want to risk getting infected. I was really scared of the disease. But I slowly got over my fear and realized that it's a lot harder to get AIDS than you might think.

I've been a nurse about seventeen years, and the first eleven of them were in hospitals. One thing that was difficult for me is that originally I worked in home care and hospice. So I'd go to one house and teach about diabetes or congestive failure — doing all this in the cure mode. I'd leave that house, drive halfway across the city and at the next place it was just about providing comfort. I was going back and forth between the cure mode and the comfort mode, and it was difficult to keep the patients straight. Years ago when I was involved in the cure side, I thought that the essence of nursing was to be able to get there when somebody was dead and bring them back with the right combination of medicine and procedures. Now that I'm in hospice, I've learned that actually it's more difficult to get someone peacefully over that border into death than it is to bring them back. Bringing them back is easy. It's getting them across, without the pain, without the anxiety, without the multiple problems, that's really hard.

Kevin was a patient of mine in 1989 who made a deep impression on me. The reason he made an impression is that he was the only AIDS patient I've ever worked with who asked me if I was gay. And I'm not gay, but to this day I've never had another patient ask me that. I had to ask Kevin, "Why does that make any difference to you?" He said, "Well, it doesn't really make any difference to me, but I'm just wondering how somebody who's not gay can act so compassionately to people that are."

That really made me think, "How am I responding to my patients? Am I focusing on the fact that they're gay or they may have been IV drug users?" And I realized something I'd never noticed before, and that was that I'd never asked how they got AIDS. I'd never asked, "Did you shoot drugs or are you gay? What nasty thing did you do to get this virus?" And I thought that if I could keep the attitude that it didn't matter how they got it, just that they had it, I'd be able to deal with them on that compassionate basis.

THE NURSE

...plays... pivotal role in the care provided by the hospice team, serving as case manager or team captain for her patients. Says... coordinating the services of other team members. A hospice nurse working full-time may service/case manage anywhere from seven to fourteen dying patients and families, depending on the agency's structure, the driving distances between homes, and the patients' intensity of need. Nurses prescribe and carry out their own schedules and are responsible for visiting every patient on their caseload on a regular basis, usually at least once a week, more often when necessary. Between visits, frequent telephone contact is main...

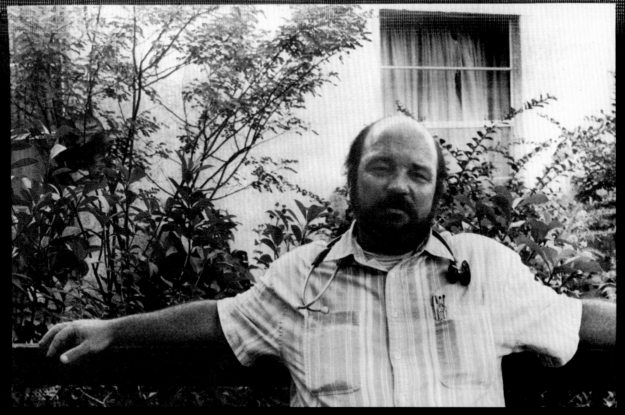

San Antonio AIDS Foundation:
Pat Day in the Foundation Garden, 1995

Interview with Sharen and Robert Rupp

Sharen: That's our son, Robby. He was a female impersonator . . . Joan Rivers. He won the local Joan Rivers look-alike contest and went to California. And we're very proud of him. We went to all his shows. He was twenty-eight when he died on December 1, 1990, World AIDS Day.

Robert: He always had a small flair for things.

Sharen: He died at three-twenty in the morning. He was coherent up to the last five or six hours. That afternoon he was in and out of a coma. His big number was "New York, New York." So I put on one of the tapes of his show, and when "New York, New York" came on he performed his last performance in bed for me. About ten that night he went into a coma and didn't come out. All of his friends were there. Bob and I were there. I curled up in bed with him and held him. He died at home. He was enrolled at Santa Rosa Hospice. Pat Day was the nurse who took care of him.

Robert: He had over four hundred and fifty people at his funeral. So he did something with his life.

Sharen: The procession to the cemetery was a mile and a half long; he'd have been proud. And it wasn't your normal funeral. After the service was over, while people filed out, we had "New York, New York" playing in the background. His stage name was Courtney Rose. We had a bunch of single roses, and everybody came by and picked up a rose and laid it inside the casket.

Sharen Rupp became the director of the San Antonio AIDS Foundation in October 1991. She passed away in the fall of 1995 from a heart attack.

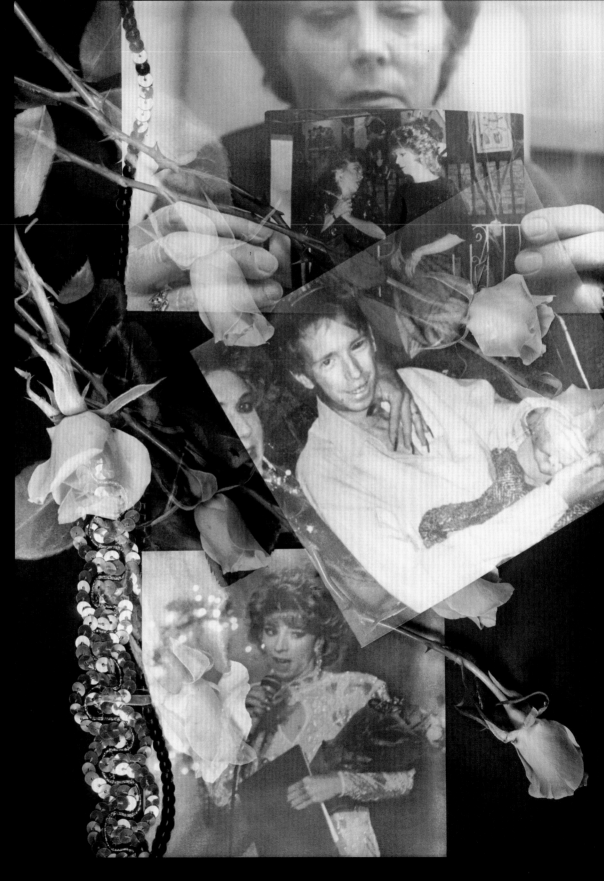

San Antonio AIDS Foundation:

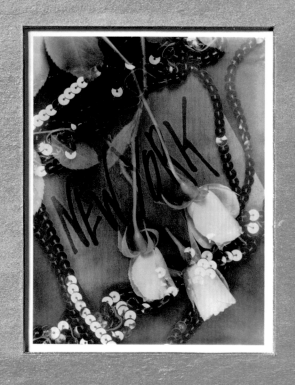

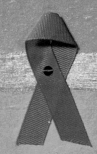

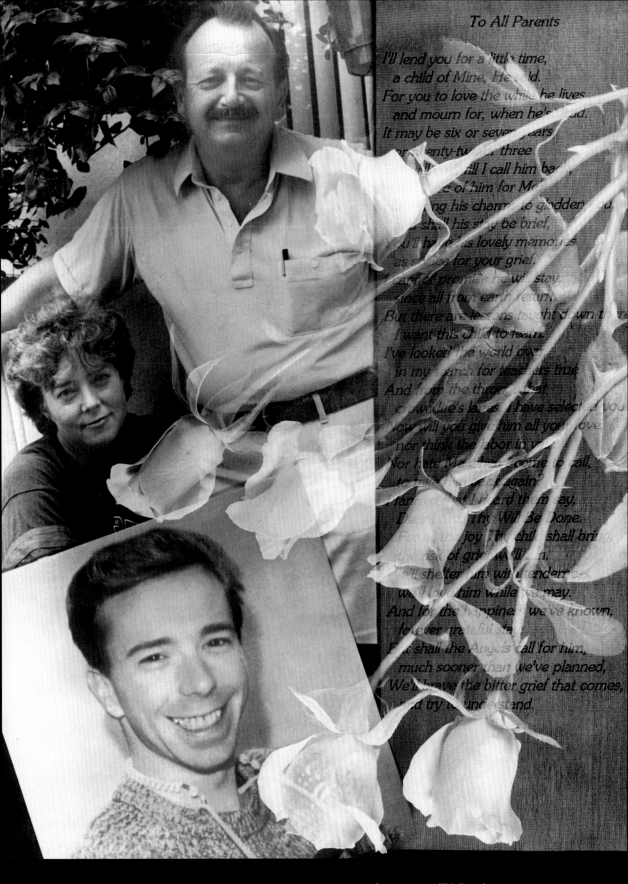

To All Parents

I'll lend you for a little time,
   a child of Mine, He said.
For you to love the while he lives
   and mourn for, when he's dead.
It may be six or seven years
   or twenty-two or three
But will you, till I call him back,
   take care of him for Me?
He'll bring his charms to gladden you,
   and shall his stay be brief,
You'll have his lovely memories
   as solace for your grief.
I cannot promise he will stay,
   since all from earth return,
But there are lessons taught down there
   I want this child to learn.
I've looked the world over
   in my search for teachers true
And from the throngs that
   crowd life's lanes I have selected you.
Now will you give him all your love,
   nor think the labor in vain,
Nor hate Me when I come to call,
   to take him back again?
I fancied that I heard them say,
   Dear Lord, Thy Will Be Done.
For all the joy Thy child shall bring,
   the risk of grief we'll run.
We'll shelter him with tenderness,
   we'll love him while we may.
And for the happiness we've known,
   forever grateful stay.
But shall the Angels call for him,
   much sooner than we've planned,
We'll brave the bitter grief that comes,
   and try to understand.

San Antonio AIDS Foundation:
Sharen and Robert Rupp in Their Garden, 1995

Hospice San Antonio, 1995
Interview with Sue Dial

Sue Dial: We've always had bereavement services for our hospice families. A part of the hospice philosophy is that we take care of the entire family, not just the person dying. Therefore, we extend our services to the family with the understanding that grief is a natural result of loss. It's part of our job to help the family move through the healing process after the family member has died. We have a commitment to the family for a year after the person dies — longer if needed.

For about the past year, I got more and more calls looking for a support group for children. I realized that children were getting lost in the grieving process. They suffer as much, have as much grief to contend with, as adults do.

Lauren [Saegert] was referred by a school nurse and a counselor. (Our brochure for this program goes not only to hospice families but to school counselors and school nurses.) The school nurse sent a brochure home with Lauren [her father died in January 1995], and her mother, Lisa, called to ask about the program.

Death is something that everyone is reluctant to talk about, but it happens to all of us. Being with families in the midst of that event and helping them adjust and walk through that experience, coaching them through the process, teaching them how to say good-bye, maybe helping them heal hurts from the past before the person dies, is a wonderful experience and a wonderful service to the community.

For two years we provided a one-day camp, a support group for children. It served a purpose and was successful, but we could see that there was a need for more long-term care. So this year, our support group was extended to six weeks so we could follow the children's progress for a longer period of time. On the last day of the program, as part of a "fun day," the children from the program released balloons with messages to their family members who had died.

Children don't express their grief the way adults do. They don't have the vocabulary. They don't fully understand what death is — not that adults understand it fully. The way children express their emotions is through games, play, drama, coloring, putting scrapbooks together.

I think that if we take more of an active part in helping children heal through grief, then we can serve a real purpose in their lives as they become adults. If they don't work through those strong, hard feelings as children, it will affect their lives as adults in a negative way. I think that in the future, more hospice work will be involved in helping children.

Sue Dial is director of the children's program at Hospice San Antonio.

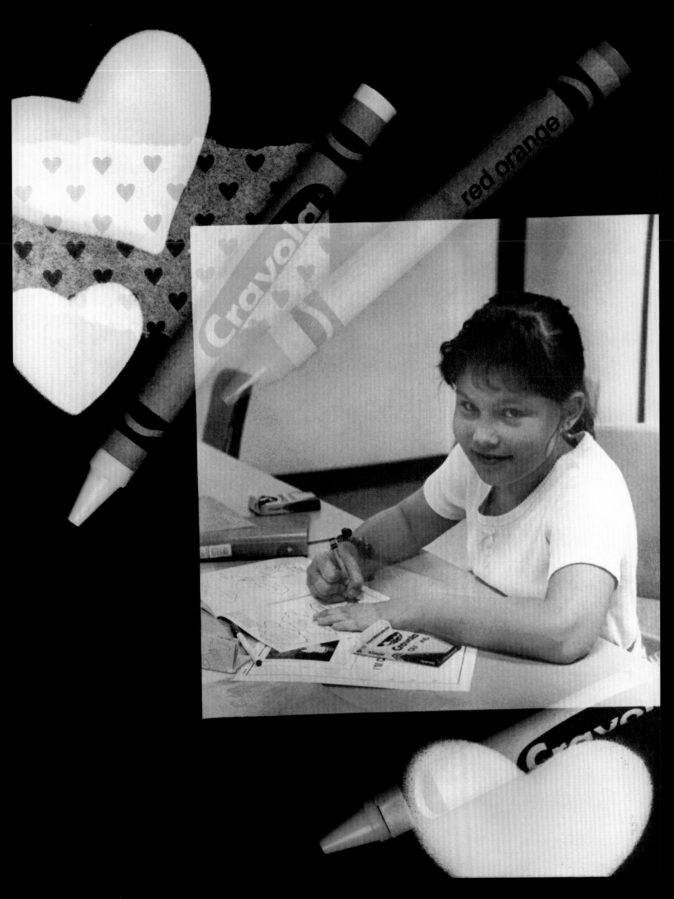

Hospice San Antonio:
Lauren Saegert, 1995

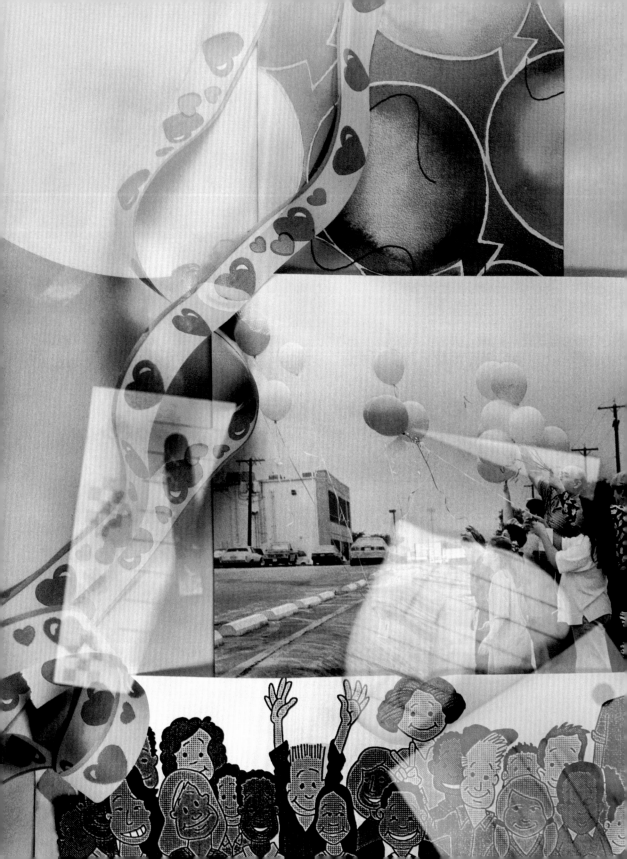

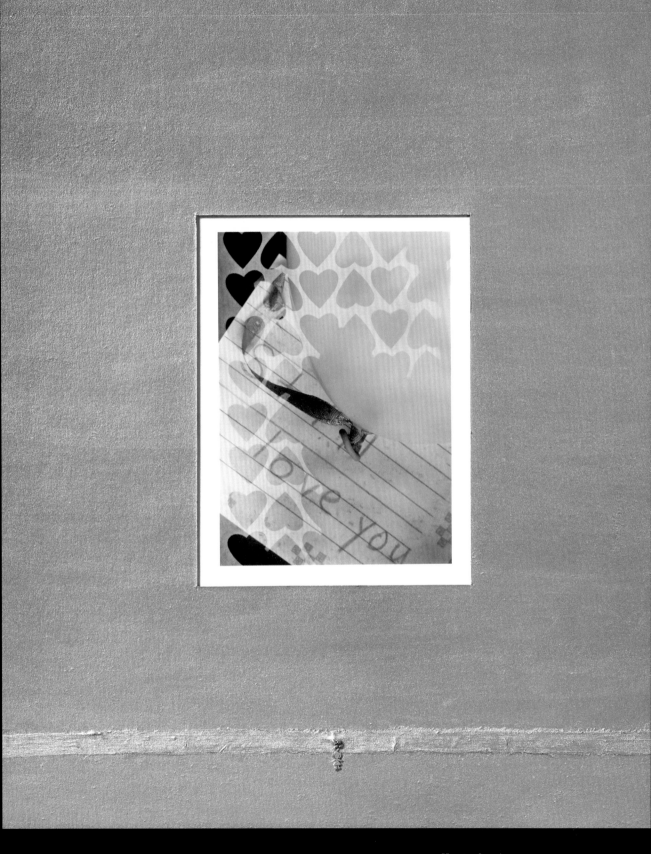

Hospice San Antonio:
Shrine for the Children's Program, 1995

Papa Day, 1994

Interviews with Donald Day Boyer, Penelope Alice Boyer, and Katherine Eleanor Boyer Reisert

Donald Day Boyer (son): Papa Day [Willard Day Boyer] was a marine in World War I; it was the big event in his life. He volunteered. He was a young man and wanted the excitement. He enlisted late in 1917; by early 1918 he was taken in a troopship to Brest, France. He saw action in the Argonne Forest. He was there only a short time before he was wounded, shot in the leg, and was in a convalescent hospital at Armistice. He was very proud of his war record and of having been wounded.

When he came back from the war, he became a pharmacist in Washington, D.C. His pharmacy was located very close to the White House. As it happened, Admiral Richard E. Byrd was in the pharmacy having a prescription filled at the time Roosevelt's death was announced. My father and he listened together, there in the pharmacy. From that day on they struck up a friendship that lasted over the years until Byrd's death. They would get together and have long conversations about the world. My father had an autographed copy of Byrd's book, *Alone,* and a lot of Byrd memorabilia. By the time my father got terminally ill in 1980, '81, Medicare had happened. In February 1981, he was sent to the VA hospital in New Haven. When he was diagnosed with terminal cancer, the VA didn't want him. He was sent to the Connecticut Hospice in Branford, which had just opened and was only ten miles from the VA. It was small but rather elegant; it was not his choice to go to a hospice, nor his family's choice, but it was a fine place for my father. He was treated very well in the hospice. All our family were very impressed with the care and sympathy he received. Much more attention was paid to him as a person.

Penelope Alice Boyer (granddaughter): He lived with us all my life. When we moved to Danbury, he lived in the apartment next door. He loved limericks. When I was a little girl we did "Louella Annabel Patricia's Birthday Party" together. It had an orchestra of insects.

Papa Day was very proud of his friendship with Admiral Richard Byrd. As Papa Day got more senile, he confused what he imagined with what had actually happened in his life. One of his "war memories" was touching both of the poles, the North Pole and the South Pole. Of course he never did this, but it had to do with his friend Admiral Byrd.

When he got sick it was very early in the hospice movement. I had never heard the word "hospice" before.

Katherine Eleanor Boyer Reisert (granddaughter): Papa must have wanted to travel in space. After he became senile he used to tell me that he remembered going to Sugarloaf Mountain and there was a launch pad there and he blasted off and went to the moon. He was wearing a big glass bowl helmet so he could breathe. I was around thirteen when I first heard this story. He would have been eighty-nine or ninety when he told it. And he thoroughly believed it was real.

When he got sick, we felt so grateful to hospice because in our home it was so hard for us to care for him physically and mentally, especially since he was senile. We were so glad that two weeks before he died he said about the hospice, "This is the nicest home I've ever had."

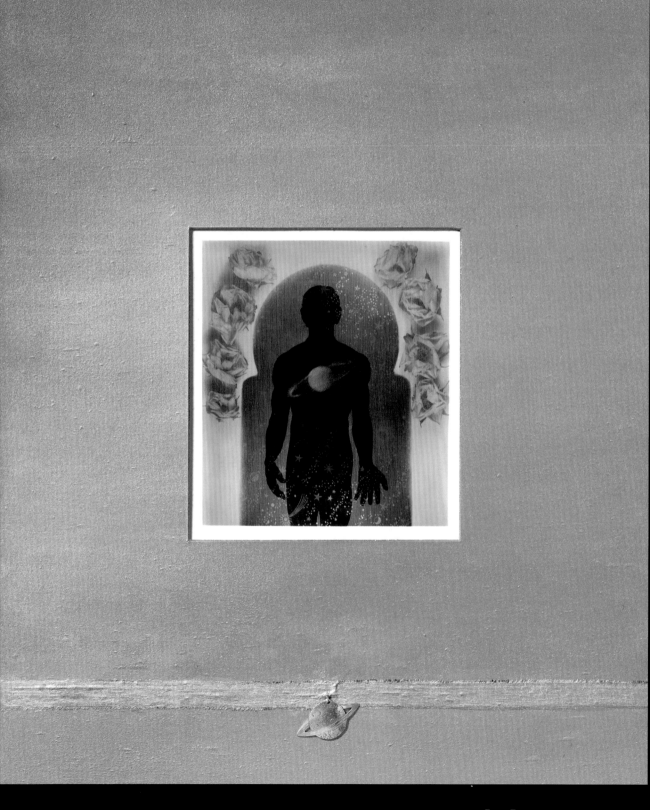

Papa Day:
Shrine for Papa Day, 1995

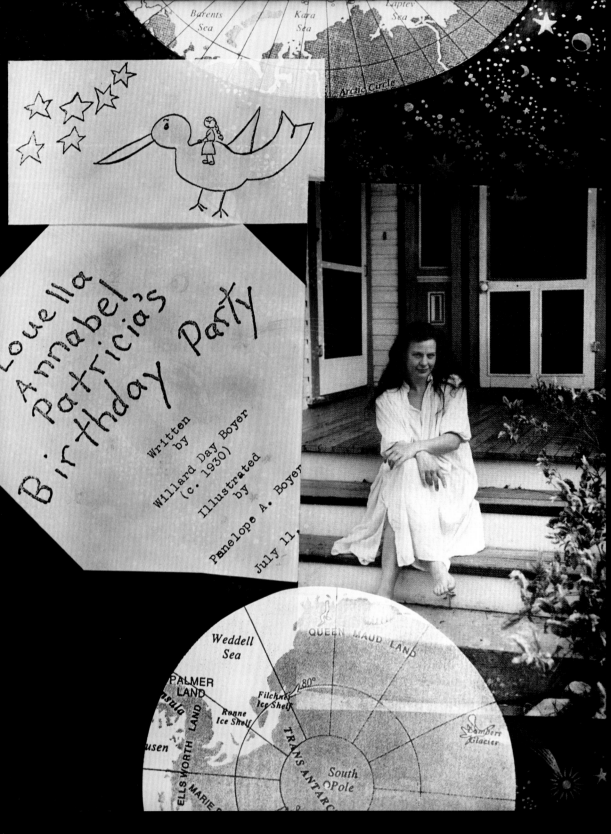

Papa Day:

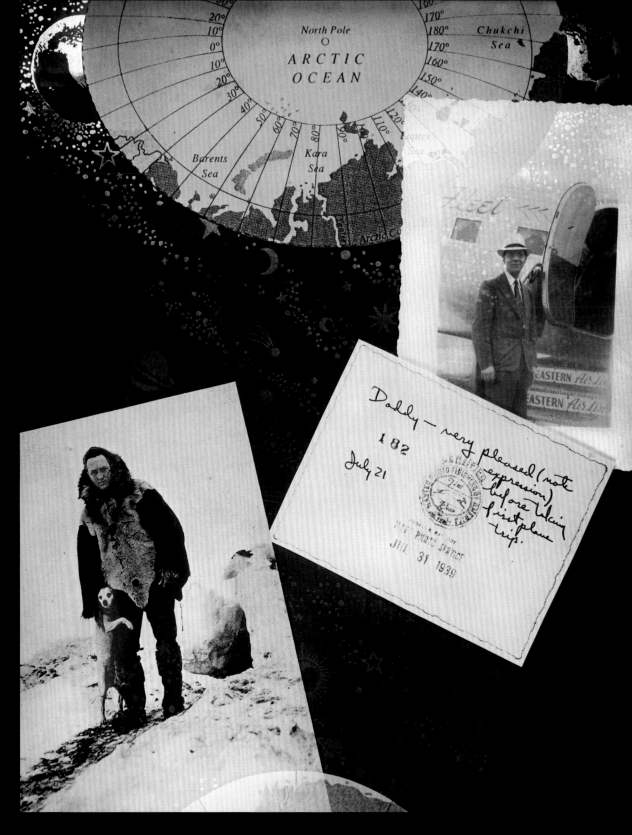

Papa Day:
Admiral Byrd with His Dog; Willard Day Boyer (Papa Day), 1995

Project Transitions, 1994

Interviews at Project Transitions, an AIDS residence in Austin, Texas, with Jason Piercy, Brandon Haga, Woody, and Cindy Lengel

Jason Piercy: I read about hospice twenty years ago, and I thought about it for a long time. I lived in Mississippi for a while and then moved back here. I had so many friends dying of AIDS in Mississippi and I couldn't be there. So I thought, "I will do this here in hopes that someone will do it for my friends there." I called Project Transitions when it was about six months old and I volunteered. In April 1989 I became the house manager. It has been a lesson for me. It makes you appreciate every moment you have. You really live that day.

Every patient here is also a patient of Hospice Austin. We're needed in the area because hospitals didn't really want AIDS patients, and the nursing homes wouldn't take them either. Yet they can't stay at home because parents aren't able to care for them or the patients are alienated from parents, although most of the time we have lots of family support.

One man had a problem with his father. He'd been rejected because he was gay. Over the years they'd built walls to keep from dealing with what had hurt them. In the last weeks, he and his father had a reconciliation. Hospice creates an atmosphere that lets everybody go to that place when they're ready. The last months of life can be one of the greatest growth experiences, and I see that a lot here.

Brandon Haga: I've been on staff six weeks; I volunteered for about four months before that. I wouldn't be here if I hadn't really had a heartfelt desire to be on staff. It's tremendous. There's so much you can learn — about yourself, about other people, about so many things — in these walls. It's these times that are making me grow as a person and making me feel like I'm contributing something.

We don't really refer to these folks as patients. They're residents. This is their house; this is their home. That's what hospice is all about. Mostly it's just a big family with other relatives that visit at times.

Woody: I've been here about a month. My family visits me very frequently. They live nearby. They brought me here so I'd be close, so they could visit me. I'm not in condition anymore to live on my own and my parents work, so this was the logical answer. You pretty well feel like you're in a house. All these things are mine. That's one of my dogs; he's a pug. I collect fairies. When my ex-lover and I were still living together, we had a Victorian living room. We had put angels all over it. Then I was redoing the dining room and decided that I didn't want it to be the same. So I bought fairies, which are a lot harder to find.

Cindy Lengel: I had a friend who was a volunteer at Omega House, another AIDS house in Austin, and she used to tell me about the strong spiritual experiences she witnessed in working with people with AIDS. And I wanted that. So I chose to be here because of the spirituality it offered. Because of being here, I've changed my mind about how people operate, what their needs are, what my needs are. We're more spiritual than physical. It's easier to take care of people physically and not so easy to meet their spiritual needs.

When I think of the residents I've met here, I see a flood of faces; each person brings with them a lifetime of experiences. They come here incapacitated, so they can't be themselves as they were before AIDS. I remember Larry. We called him "caretaker." He was here for a while and took care of the garden and the cats. Then his family took him back home. In the meantime he'd gotten attached to one of our kittens, Nicky. Toward the end, Larry was very anxiety-ridden; he was afraid. It was hard to watch that; hard to accept. He wasn't having the kind of death I wanted for him. He was having a hard time letting go. I knew Larry was ready to go when he asked Jason to keep and take care of Nicky, when he gave Nicky back to us.

Jason Piercy is House Manager of Project Transitions. Cindy Lengel is Volunteer Coordinator.

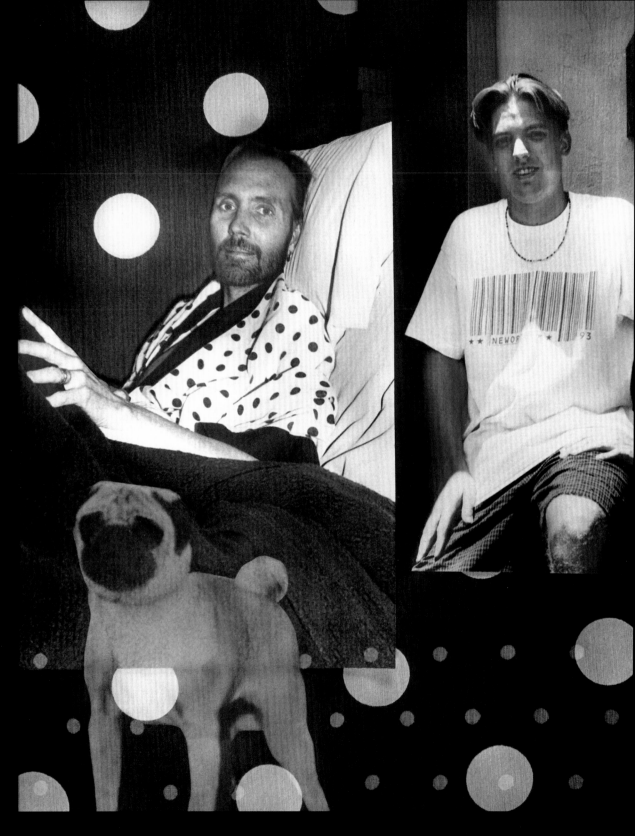

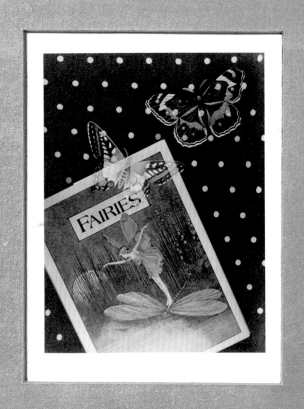

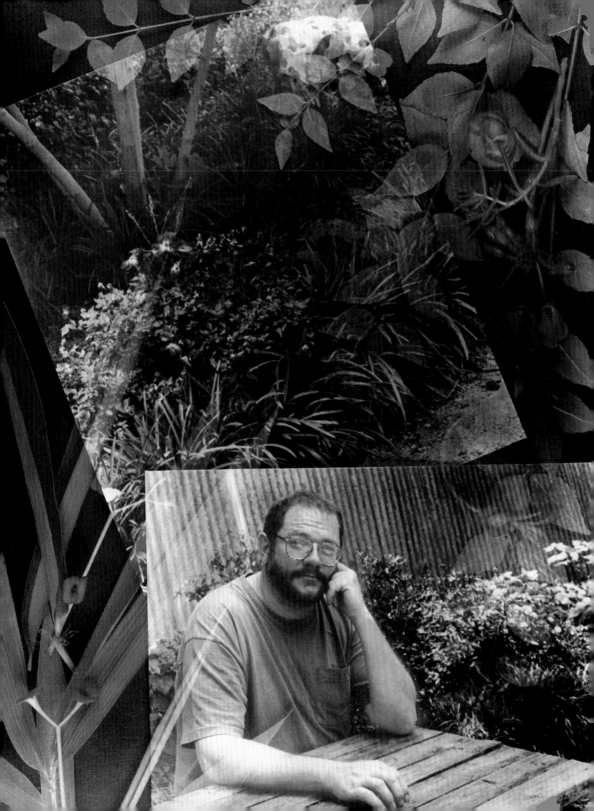

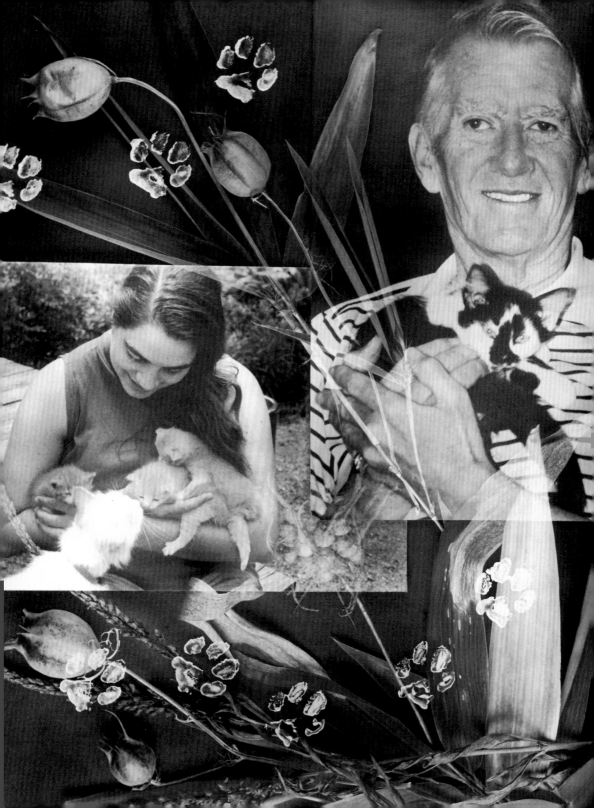

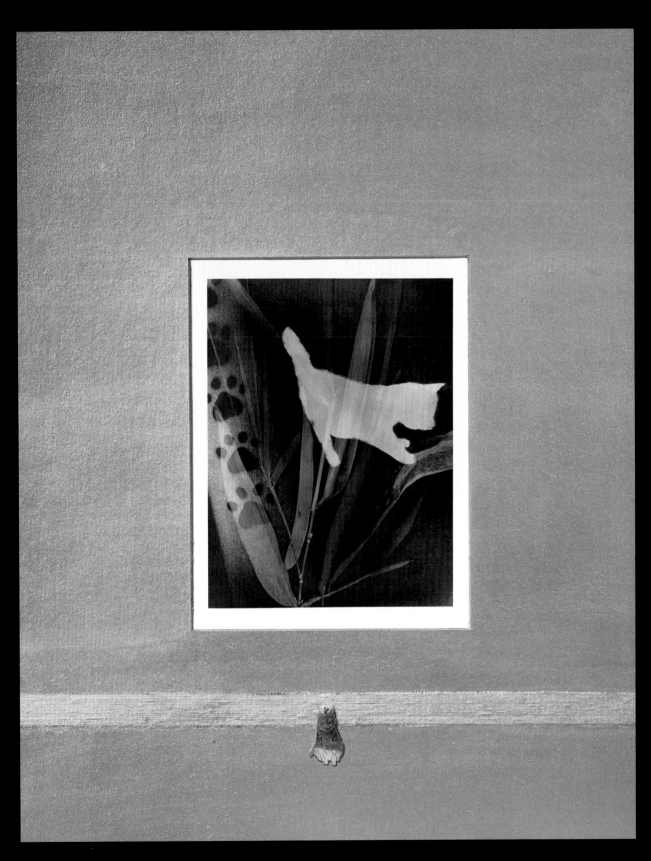

Project Transitions:
Shrine for Larry, 1994

The Yatteaus, 1994

Interview with Jack and Vivian Yatteau about Jack's uncle, Edward Richard Levy, and Vivian's mother, Marian Suchards, both of whom received hospice care

Jack: My uncle Edward was my mother's brother, the youngest of four children. I grew up with Ed. My parents separated, and I lived with my mother and her family. Ed was a combination of older brother and father. He taught me so many things: how to roller skate; how to swim and dive; how to throw a baseball. We shared a bedroom.

When I was seven, he left to go to college and I really missed him. He went to Vermont University in his first year and was active in the National Guard. That's where he had his first exposure to military life. Then he transferred to Columbia College in New York City. From there he went to Columbia Law School.

When the war broke out, he volunteered for the infantry. He was assigned to the Tenth Armored Division, Twentieth Armored Infantry Battalion, which served in Europe during World War II. He was at the south end of the Battle of the Bulge, and I was at the northern end. He won a Purple Heart and a Bronze Star.

After the war he practiced real estate law.

He was diagnosed with prostate cancer about eight years before he died. He had a very bad last year. He was constantly in the hospital being treated. Then they couldn't do any more. He went to a hospice — Hospice by the Sea, Inc. — then he came home and died in his own surroundings.

The main thing about hospice was that it gave his wife, Gladys, some rest. She was at her wit's end. She was constantly taking care of him. She couldn't get any rest, night or day. While he was in the hospice, she could be there during the day, then go home at night and rest. She was there every day.

Vivian: Hospice always meant hospital to me. But then we went to visit him, and it was beautiful. His accommodations were wonderful.

My mother, Marian Suchards, came to the United States from Austria with her mom, her two sisters, and two younger brothers when she was seven.

Throughout her life my mother worked. She learned sewing from my grandmother, who was a very skilled seamstress who had her own business. One of her jobs was with Rudolph Gowns in New York. Rudolph used to make Eleanor Roosevelt's dresses — her formal dresses — and Kate Smith's. I think mother even met them. She was in charge of finishing, to see that the gowns were in perfect condition before they were sent out. She had a beautiful dress made for me — burgundy velvet — which I styled. I wanted a princess style with covered buttons down the back, long sleeves, a scooped neck. Those memories are going to keep flooding back. I hadn't thought about that dress in years.

She said something to me at one point, with her lips trembling: "If I've ever hurt you in any way. . . ." That brought tears to my eyes. She actually asked my forgiveness.

She was diagnosed with pancreatic cancer. She was at a beautiful hospice (Hospice of Martin, Inc.). It looked like a private residence on the outside. The day my mother arrived, they were fixing the room up for her and I saw that they had their linen room stacked high with handmade afghans, all made by volunteers.

Mother acclimated beautifully. She loved the attention and the care. The residence worked for us because she didn't want anyone in the house but she needed someone around.

My mother died peacefully in her sleep on November 20, 1994. She was ninety-six and a half years old.

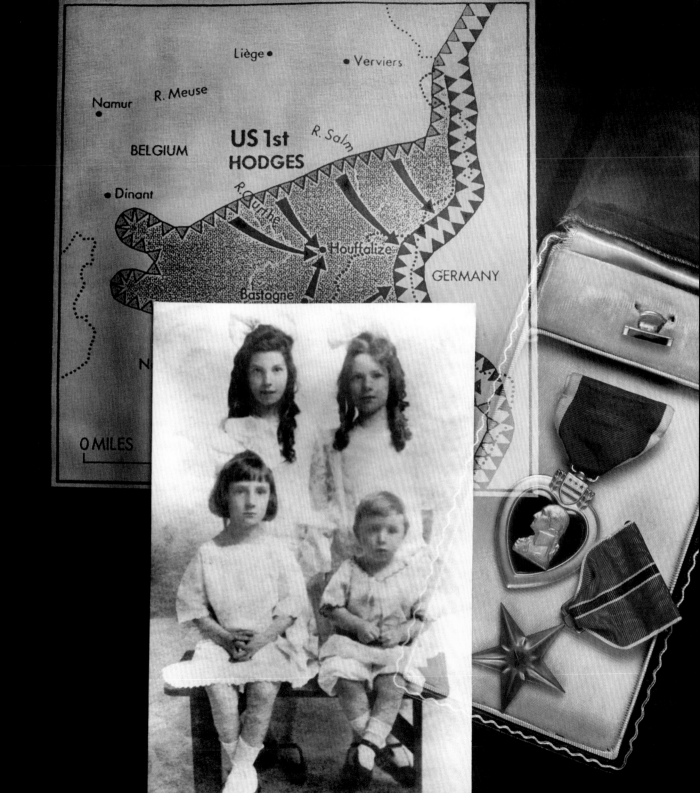

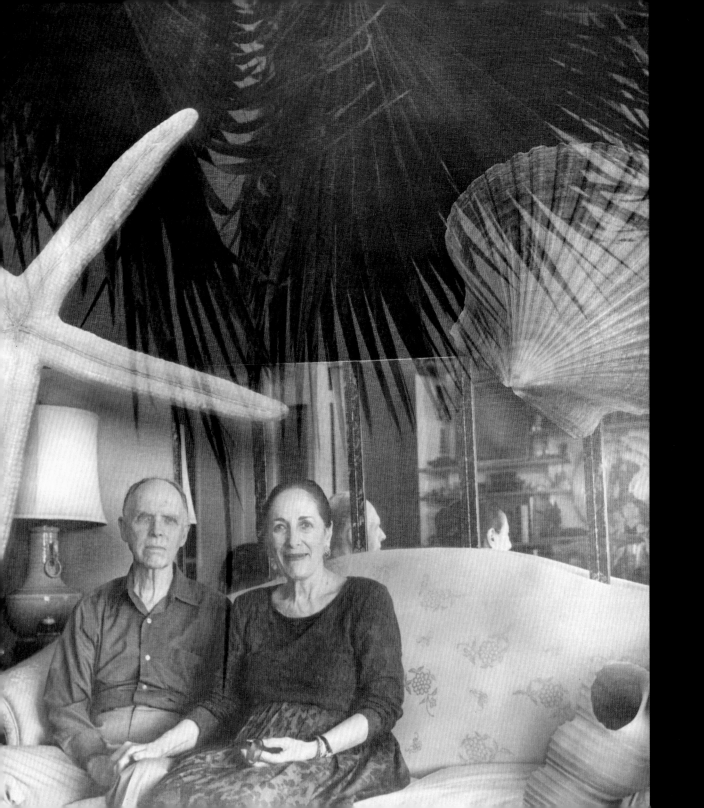

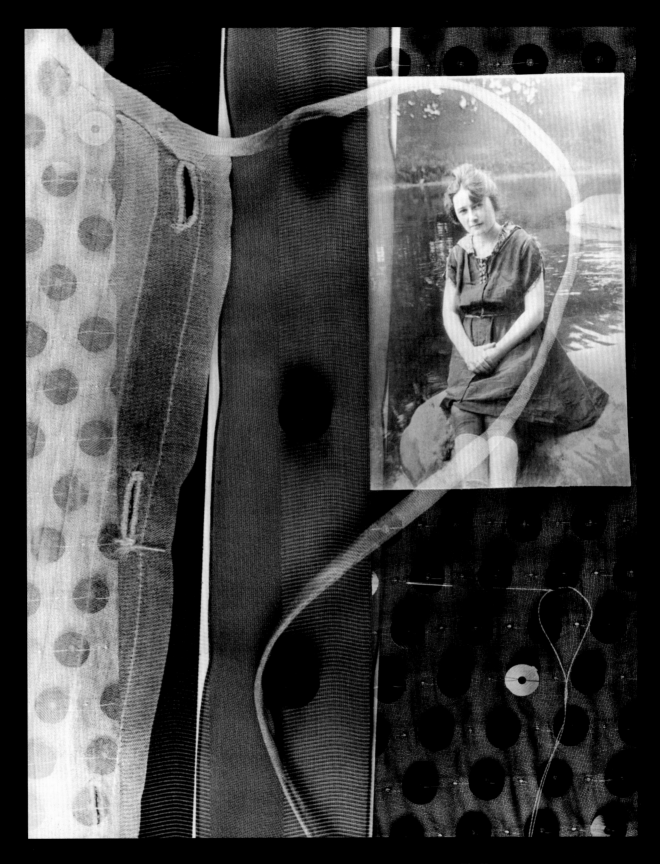

The Yatteaus:
Marian Suchards, 1994

HOSPICE ON FILM: Three Stories
Interview with Susan Froemke, Deborah Dickson, and Albert Maysles
by Philip Brookman

A documentary film about hospice was commissioned by Home Box Office for national broadcast at the time of the opening of *Hospice: A Photographic Inquiry*. This film, produced and directed by Susan Froemke, Deborah Dickson, and Albert Maysles of Maysles Films, Inc., is also included in the exhibition. It tells of three terminally ill patients and their families, and the impact of hospice care on their diverse experiences.

Susan Froemke, a four-time Emmy Award–winner, is an advocate of "direct cinema." She has completed fourteen nonfiction films, including *Ozawa, Christo in Paris, Vladimir Horowitz: The Last Romantic, Baroque Duet, Soldiers of Music: Rostropovich Returns to Russia,* and *Abortion: Desperate Choices.* Deborah Dickson began her long-term collaboration with Maysles Films, Inc., after studying filmmaking at New York University. Her own films include the Academy Award–nominated *Stetloff: Memoirs of a Bookseller,* and *Sex, Teens, and Public Schools.* Her work with Maysles Films, Inc., includes *Christo in Paris* and *Abortion: Desperate Choices.* Albert Maysles, with his brother David, is recognized as an architect of "direct cinema," a style of documentary filmmaking that relies on the unobstructed observation and organization of events rather than the use of scripts and narration to tell stories. His films include *Salesman, Gimme Shelter, Grey Gardens,* and *Valley Curtain.*

I spoke to Froemke, Dickson, and Maysles before their new film was completed, and they asked to begin with a poem by thirteenth-century mystic Jelaluddin Rumi, which they learned while shooting at Home Hospice of Sonoma:

> *The way of love is not*
> *a subtle argument.*
> *The door there*
> *is devastation.*
> *Birds make great sky-circles*
> *of their freedom.*
> *How do they learn it?*
> *They fall, and falling,*
> *they're given wings.*

Jelaluddin Rumi, from *Birdsong*, translated by Coleman Barks

Susan Froemke, Deborah Dickson, and Albert Maysles
Hospice patient Michael Merseal, Jr. with his father and mother, Missoula, Montana, 1995

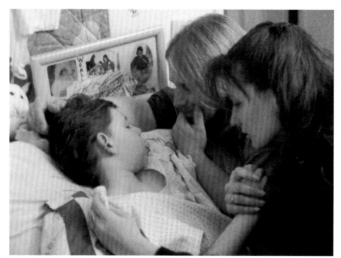

Philip Brookman: Describe your film about hospice.

Susan Froemke: Our film interweaves three stories, each about a hospice patient and his or her family. The first, shot in Missoula, Montana, is about eight-year-old Michael Merseal, who lies comatose on his living room couch in the final stages of an incurable brain disease. Yet, he changes the lives of all who knew him. His mother has abandoned the family, his father has quit work to care for him, and his nine-year-old sister is trying to deal with the loss of her mother and brother. Michael seems to hang on to life through months of silence, until his mother finally appears. Only then is he able to die, peacefully, between his parents.

Deborah Dickson: The second part is about Anna Turner, a forty-six-year-old African-American woman in Queens who is dying of lung cancer at home surrounded by her family: her mother and two children. Her son, the only one still at home, is seventeen. Her daughter, a Marine, has come with her child to help care for Anna. Anna is a very religious woman — a fundamentalist — who believes that if she prays every day and thanks God for healing her, she will be completely cured. She feels that her work on earth is not complete, and dreams of becoming a minister. Anna's faith gives her strength and joy, but at the same time prevents her from doing the end-of-life work that hospice believes is so productive. Anna cannot accept that she's dying and at the same time have faith that she is being healed by God. According to her pastor, this type of "doublemindedness" nullifies her prayer. Anna gets one wish. Her pain is well managed by hospice care, and she is able to remain at home. She isn't cured, but her faith is unshaken until the last hours of her life, leaving her son unprepared for his loss. When the hospice chaplain asks him to say good-bye and give his mother permission to go, he can't. He asks, "What was all the praying for?" His questions are those we all have, such as: why does someone we love and need have to die?

SF: The third story, set in Sonoma County, California, is about sixty-two-year-old Ralph Armstrong, who lies in a rehab center, partially paralyzed by a fatal brain tumor. Only a few weeks before he became ill, he was backpacking in the mountains. Now, facing imminent death, he has fallen into despair. Yet, his hospice doctor and chaplain believe that, given the chance to resolve deeply eroded family relationships, he may be on the threshold of a transformation.

DD: Ralph is a man who has been totally out of touch with his feelings, and now he's able to cry for the first time in fifty years. The possibility of spiritual transformation is the core of his story. But in order for such transformation to take place, one needs to go through despair, and it's very helpful if there's someone to "accompany" you on that difficult and lonely journey. Ralph's story interested me because, as Home Hospice of Sonoma's CEO, True Ryndes, points out, there are so many deaths we experience throughout our lives, such as deaths of ego or identity. Once we've been through that sort of experience, we learn to put things together again. I think this helps us to face death when it comes, or at least helps us not to succumb to the chaos and despair that can accompany it.

SF: This concept — the "potential for grace" at the end of one's life — surprised me, and I find it very reassuring. It's all about being able to let go of the constraints that have bound you throughout

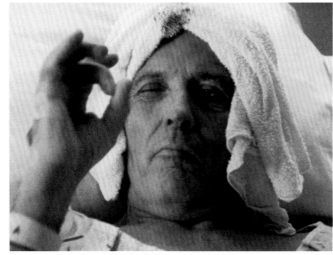

Susan Froemke, Deborah Dickson, and Albert Maysles
Hospice patient
Ralph Armstrong,
Sonoma, California, 1995

your life and about letting go and allowing yourself to fall into the unknown. It's a step toward spiritual growth, and with the help of a skilled hospice team it can sometimes lead to a powerful, personal transformation. It's this type of hospice philosophy that I find helpful and that I hope will be of use to others, especially those who flinch when the subject of death comes up.

Albert Maysles: I've had so many deaths in my family that now I don't cry quite so much. But I remain deeply touched by the darker personal truths that seem to emerge, especially when people are faced with death and dying. In every story of our film, society's and each person's veil of denial reveals very soulful elements of humanity that you don't experience in daily life. When this happens, you identify very closely with, and become fond of, each family member. For example, you understand Ralph's wife's anger and frustration over his closed emotions, yet you know there's no way he can open up. In one tiny moment when he does, you're pulling for him all the way. On the other hand, Michael's silence and his family's rapt attentiveness and love make you ponder the power of the unspoken. I can see Michael dying in his mother's arms. The image is just like the Pietà. It surprised me that, because Anna was such a loving and devoted person, I could respect her religious views without accepting them for myself. It's odd that, in our noisy and distracting world, it's only when face-to-face with death that we experience what is often missing in life: a sense of community, of lost opportunities, of the healing effect of painful memories. Hospice workers know all this, which may be why their work is more satisfying than grim.

PB: How do you translate these feelings to film?

AM: You have to be very patient, not judgmental or artificial. It's full of surprises. That's what makes a film real.

SF: Doing this project, our expectations were constantly changing. For example, this child who was silent all his life was probably waiting to hear his mother's voice again. He needed that sense of completion before he could die. Unexpectedly, she arrived at his home, and he died very quickly once he heard her say she loved him. And then, of course, the mother's grief was monumental.

DD: It's like a Greek tragedy, so deep and profound. Michael's mother was totally unprepared to face the death of her child. There was so much left unresolved. Often those who have the worst relationship with a dying person take it the hardest, because there's so much left undone.

PB: Was Michael trying to reconcile his parents' relationship through his silence?

SF: The community, the hospice, and the parents all attributed many qualities to this child. They constantly were calling him "the Christ child." You walked into that house, you knelt down by the couch where he was dying, and it was like a manger. There were stuffed animals all around him. Even though the hospice was trying to orchestrate the best passing for him — with family and friends around — you felt like the child was also orchestrating something. He had his mother and father there together at the end, and one hoped that some of the pain and conflict between them would be healed. Here is this child who can't walk or talk — never could — but in many ways he is a great teacher. A lot of love surrounded him and he brought value into people's lives.

PB: Has your understanding of hospice changed through this project?

SF: I worked out some of my own fears relating to death, a subject I had totally avoided. I didn't know what hospice was before this film. I thought it was some place — like a house — where you went to die. My own parents are elderly and I was anxious about having to face their eventual death. I would shut down whenever I thought about it because the images I associated with dying — to be in a hospital bed, in a sterile environment, where your family comes in only at certain hours — seemed so painful. It seemed so lonely to be all by yourself at the end. The medical profession is not trained to deal with dying. They're trained to heal on a physical, rather than spiritual, level. What I learned from hospice is that it doesn't have to be that way at all. There are alternatives.

DD: For me, and I hope for others, this is also a wake-up call: to appreciate life, even in its small, ordinary moments; to not take health for granted; to resolve relationships; to express deep feelings; to live as fully as possible; and to not wait until I am dying to realize what's important about living.

PB: Your style of filmmaking furthers our understanding of the characters through an accumulation of details. How does this work?

DD: Much of the power of film is in the richness of details rather than in the ideas that drive the story. For example, Anna had the most beautifully manicured, polished red nails. One day, a hospice worker said, "You must be feeling better today. I notice your nails are done." Anna looked up and said, "Vanity takes no vacation."

SF: That moment really made us laugh. Anna's wit is so sweet and fetching that this detail makes you fall in love with her. As you start to love Anna, you realize you don't want her to die. You're emotionally connected and for the rest of the film you experience the feeling of seeing a loved one slip away.

PB: In this way, have you been able to discover something true about these people in your film, or document the truth of their experiences?

AM: Because it's reality that governs us in filming, it helps enormously in keeping you honest. We can't control events, nor do we want to. Sure, we're only human, so we have points of view. But they can be put at a distance. All of this leaves our subjects free to be themselves.

SF: We don't have control over what our subjects do. We spend a lot of time with them, so we get to know them intimately. Many people feel that you tamper with the environment by going into it with a camera and sound equipment. We really attempt not to interfere or change what's happening. But you still have to develop a real connection with your subjects. The question is, "How do you do that without tampering in some way?"

DD: Of course we're changing the environment in some way. We're there with cameras, and people are self-conscious. But I think that the trust we develop with our subjects counterbalances the impact of our presence.

SF: We discovered early on in the filming that what happened during the last days and hours of a person's life is the most unpredictable. Firm beliefs often unraveled, allowing unexpected healing. And so, we most wanted to be present to film during these hours. Also, to my knowledge, these types of scenes had never been filmed intimately before. So it was quite a challenge. The trust between you and your subject

Susan Froemke, Deborah Dickson, and Albert Maysles
Pentecostal priest Bishop George with hospice patient Anna Turner, Queens, New York, 1995

has to be extremely tight because of this intimacy. You become part of the life-experience of your dying subjects. You are one of the last images they see in their lives. They must invite you to participate, to be a witness. We were fortunate to establish relationships with the patients and their families that enabled us to draw a portrait of their final days. They felt it was valuable to let others see their experiences and the good work that hospice does.

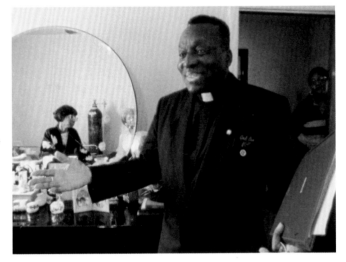

AM: Yeah, the work we do is important to the subjects. Of course, it's important to the filmmaker, but it's also important to the subjects that their stories be told. When our subjects see the final film, there is instant verification.

PB: Are you memorializing these people?

SF: Yes, in a sense. Anna knew that she would be memorialized in some way. She understood this more than her family did. She always wanted us to be there because I think she wanted everyone to be of strong faith, and she communicated this through the film. However, the hospice concept is not just about preserving memories. At Home Hospice of Sonoma, where Ralph was a patient, a lot of energy is spent on psychological counseling. Dr. Brad Stuart, the medical director, talks about how a dying person's illness can burn away his persona, allowing him a glimpse of his inner core, his true self. There's tremendous value in this process if you can get through it and transform yourself, even if it happens just for a few minutes before death. The peace you attain through this process can affect your family and those you're close to. This can engender profound feelings that may reverberate for generations. But what do you strive for? Is it peace? Is it acceptance?

DD: It's about connecting to your soul.

PB: Did you find that you can film death or represent it in some way on film?

AM: You can ask, "Could we — should we — have made this film on such a taboo subject?" Well, we did it thanks to the openness and courage of our subjects. It's so important and long overdue.

HOSPICE CARE TODAY

From time to time I am asked whether people shy away from discussing the option of hospice care with their family member, loved one, or patient because, for some, hospice care might represent "giving up hope." The answer is yes, some people, including professional health-care providers, do resist talking about the availability and appropriateness of hospice care for a terminally ill person because, to them, hospice care is about death and giving up hope. One of the goals of the National Hospice Foundation and its sister organization, the National Hospice Organization, in organizing and supporting the photographic exhibition captured in this book is to portray the true philosophy of hospice care. The hospice philosophy emphasizes life, not death. And, while "hope for a miracle cure" may not be evident in hospice philosophy, hospice care can be an extraordinary expression of hope and individual courage.

Hope in hospice care is represented in the day-to-day value of life of the patients and families using hospice care: the autonomy and control exercised by the individual in the hospice environment, the ability to be free from pain on a daily basis, the ability to be in his or her own home or in a homelike environment, the ability to reflect upon one's life and to come to and experience closure with loved ones.

Last year, hospices across the country cared for approximately 340,000 patients and families. Most of these patients were over the age of sixty-five, with a diagnosis of cancer; however, almost 40 percent were under the age of sixty-five, and many (approximately 15 percent) had diseases other than cancer. Most hospices require that a patient have a life-limiting prognosis. To be eligible for hospice benefits under Medicare, Medicaid, and many commercial insurance plans, a patient must have a prognosis of six months or less, if the disease were to run a "normal" course.

When selecting hospice care, patients and families are participating in a unique experience beginning with the fact that they choose hospice care after a process of "informed consent." A patient cannot be forced into hospice care, and some people, for their own respected and individual reasons, may choose not to receive hospice care.

When a patient and family select hospice care, they can expect to receive a responsive, coordinated, comprehensive set of services from a team of hospice professionals including physician and nursing services, in-patient and respite care, home health aide services, physical and other therapies, social work and counseling services, and spiritual care such as assistance in working with local clergy. The hospice program also provides assistance in arranging for medications, supplies, and medical equipment. These services are coordinated through a patient's personal plan of care, and although the disease is clearly recognized in developing the plan of care, the goal is to care for the patient and family, not to treat the disease.

Most hospice patients have their own doctor, who must agree to the use of hospice care, and the hospice program encourages the active involvement of this physician as part of the hospice team. If the patient does not have his or her own physician, the hospice doctor provides the necessary medical services. The hospice physician is also available to provide consultation to other physicians on such issues as pain and symptom control, as necessary.

Another important member of the team is the volunteer. Every hospice patient/family is offered a volunteer to be of assistance to the patient and family during this time. Other hospice volunteers work in the office, on fund-raising committees and on the boards of hospices. The NHO estimates that of the 115,000 persons involved with hospice care across the country, 95,000 are volunteers. Every year these volunteers give more than five million hours to helping dying persons and their families. I would encourage people interested in being a hospice volunteer to contact a hospice program in their community.

Hospice care is usually provided in the patient's own residence; occasionally the patient's home may be a group home or a nursing home. Hospice care is usually provided on an intermittent basis, meaning that the hospice nurse may visit one or more times a week, usually for an hour or two, based on the needs of the patient. Other hospice staff also visit on an intermittent basis, depending on the patient's need and plan of care. This usually requires that a responsible person be available to provide care to the patient when the hospice personnel and volunteers are not with the patient. This caregiver is usually a family member, but can also be a friend, a volunteer, or a paid attendant.

Another unique aspect of hospice care is the availability of bereavement care for the family following the death of the patient. Bereavement support varies according to the needs of the individual and may involve occasional contact from the hospice staff and volunteers, participation in support groups, or referral to individual counselors.

Hospice care is a covered benefit under most private and public health plans. Medicare provides a hospice benefit to the approximately 37 million Medicare beneficiaries. This benefit was first extended to Medicare beneficiaries in 1983 and it is estimated that more than 200,000 terminally ill Medicare beneficiaries chose hospice care in 1994. Under Medicare, the hospice program is paid directly for all services the patient needs, including professional services, on a per diem basis. The beneficiary is charged little or nothing for these services, as the hospice program is "at risk" for the cost of the care. If the cost of care is greater than what Medicare is paying the hospice, the hospice will make up the difference since it is not allowed to reduce required services, nor charge the patient. The per diem method of payment to the hospice is calculated in such a manner that the hospice program should come close to breaking even at the end of the year; however, many hospices must raise money to reach this point and to provide those important extra services that make hospice the very special care for which it is recognized across the nation.

The recent increase in awareness and interest in end-of-life issues, as demonstrated by the proliferation of articles and television programs incorporating hospice care, suggests that people are concerned about the way they will die. The experience of hospice team members tells us that people do not fear death as much as they fear dying in pain, dying alone, being a burden on their family, and being denied the dignity with which they lived their lives.

Hospice pledges to the patient that the hospice will do everything necessary to keep the patient pain-free, that the patient will not be abandoned, and that the hospice will work tirelessly to ease the patient's suffering. Hospice understands that caring for a terminally ill person at home is hard work, and the hospice will be there, every step of the way, to ease the burden on the patient and family. The hospice also promises to respect the dignity of the patient so that the dying process can be an opportunity for meaningful communication and growth.

This opportunity was most eloquently summarized by a young hospice patient who said, "They [hospice] cannot add days to your life, but they can absolutely add life to your days."

John J. Mahoney
President
National Hospice Foundation
and National Hospice Organization

The National Hospice Foundation (NHF) is headquartered in Arlington, Virginia. Its mission is to raise funds and support projects related to hospice education and research. The National Hospice Organization (NHO) is a membership organization, also headquartered in Virginia, with a mission to be an advocate for the needs of the terminally ill. For more information about hospice care or to locate a hospice program in your area, you may write the NHO at 1901 North Moore, Suite 901, Arlington, Virginia 22209, or call 1-800-658-8898.

GENERAL

Appleton, Michael, M.D., and Todd Henschell. *At Home with Terminal Illness*. New Jersey: Prentice Hall, 1995.

Bayley, Joseph. *The Last Thing We Talk About: Help and Hope for Those Who Grieve*. Elgin, Ill.: Life Journey Books, 1992.

Beattie, Melody. *A Reason to Live*. Wheaton, Ill.: Tyndale House Publishers, 1991.

Beresford, Larry, *The Hospice Handbook: A Complete Guide*. Boston: Little, Brown and Co., 1993.

Blau, Eric. *Common Heroes: Facing a Life Threatening Illness*. Pasadena, Calif.: New Sage Press, 1989.

Bockelman, Wilfred. *Finding the Right Words: Offering Care and Comfort When You Don't Know What to Say*. Minneapolis: Augsburg Fortress, 1990.

Childs-Gowell, Elaine. *Good Grief Rituals: Tools for Healing*. Barrytown, New York: Station Hill Press, 1992.

Cornils, Stanley P. *The Mourning After: How to Manage Grief Wisely*. Saratoga, Calif.: R & E Publishers, 1990.

Corr, Charles A., Clyde M. Nabe, and Donna M. Corr. *Death and Dying, Life and Living*. Pacific Grove, Calif.: Brook/Cole Publishing, 1994.

D'Arcy, Paula. *When Your Friend Is Grieving: Building a Bridge of Love*. Wheaton, Ill.: H. Shaw Publishers, 1990.

Doka, Kenneth J. *Living with Life-Threatening Illness: A Guide for Individuals, Families, and Caregivers*. Lexington, Mass.: Lexington Books, 1993.

Du Boulay, Shirley. *Cicely Saunders, Founder of the Modern Hospice Movement*. New York: Amaryllis Press, 1984.

Fisher, Mary. *I'll Not Go Quietly*. New York: Scribners, 1995.

Fitzgerald, Helen. *The Mourning Handbook*. New York: Simon & Schuster, 1994.

Greenlee, Sharon. *When Someone Dies*. Atlanta: Peachtree Publishers, 1992.

Harwell, Amy. *Ready to Live — Prepared to Die*. Wheaton, Ill.: H. Shaw Publishers, 1995.

Hwang, Michael Tainchung, and Yitai Tsuei. *Hospice — Theory and Development*. 1988.

Kelley, Patricia, and Maggie Callanan. *Final Gifts: Understanding the Special Awareness, Needs, and Communications of the Dying*. New York: Simon & Schuster, 1992.

Kübler-Ross, Elisabeth. *On Death and Dying*. New York: Macmillan, 1969.

Larson, Dale. *The Helper's Journey: Working with People Facing Grief, Loss, and Life-Threatening Illness*. Champaign, Ill.: Research Press, 1993.

Leming, Michael R., and George E. Dickinson. *Understanding Dying, Death, and Bereavement*. Fort Worth: Holt, Rinehart and Winston, 1990.

LeShan, Lawrence. *Cancer as a Turning Point: A Handbook for People with Cancer, Their Families and Health Professionals*. New York: NAL-Dutton, 1990.

Littlewood, Jane. *Aspects of Grief: Bereavement in Adult Life*. New York: Routledge, 1992.

Madden, Edward F. *Carpe Diem: Enjoying Every Day with Terminal Illness*. Boston: Jones & Bartlett Publishers, 1993.

Manning, Doug. *Don't Take My Grief Away: What to Do When You Lose a Loved One*. San Francisco: Harper & Row, 1984.

Maxwell, Katie. *Bedside Manners: A Practical Guide to Visiting the Ill*. Grand Rapids, Mich.: Baker Book House, 1990.

Menten, Ted. *Gentle Closings: How to Say Goodbye to Someone You Love*. Philadelphia: Running Press, 1991.

Neimeyer, Robert, and Hannelore Wass. *Dying: Facing Facts*. New York: Taylor & Francis, 1995.

Nungessor, Lon G. *Axioms for Survivors: How to Live Until You Say Goodbye*. San Bernardino, Calif.: Borgo Press, 1990.

Rando, Therese. *Loss and Anticipatory Grief*. Lexington, Mass.: Lexington Books, 1986.

Southard, Samuel. *Death and Dying: A Bibliographical Survey*. New York: Greenwood Press, 1991.

Stoddard, Sandal. *The Hospice Movement: A Better Way of Caring for the Dying*. New York: Vintage Books, 1992.

Tagliaferre, Lewis. *Recovery from Loss: A Personalized Guide to the Grieving Process*. Deerfield Beach, Fla.: Health Communications, 1990.

Veninga, Robert. *A Gift of Hope: How We Survive Our Tragedies*. Boston: Little, Brown and Co., 1985.

Wolfelt, Alan. *Understanding Grief: Helping Yourself Heal*. Muncie, Ind.: Accelerated Development Inc., 1992.

CHILDREN AND FAMILIES

Armstrong-Dailey, A., and Sara Z. Goltzer, eds. *Hospice Care for Children*. New York: Oxford University Press, 1993.

Bramblett, John. *When Good-bye Is Forever: Learning to Live Again After the Loss of a Child*. New York: Ballantine Books, 1991.

Davidson, Glen W. *Living with Dying: A Guide for Relatives and Friends*. Minneapolis: Augsburg Fortress, 1975.

Fitzgerald, Helen. *The Grieving Child: A Parent's Guide*. New York: Simon & Schuster, 1992.

Fry, Virginia Lynn. *Part of Me Died Too*. New York: Dutton Children's Books, 1995.

Gaes, Jason. *My Book for Kids with Cancer*. Aberdeen, S.D.: Melius and Peterson Publishing, Inc., 1987.

Grollman, Earl A. *Straight Talk About Death for Teenagers: How to Cope with Losing Someone You Love*. Boston: Beacon Press, 1993.

Horne, Jo. *When Caring Becomes Caring For. . . . A Survival Guide for Family Caregivers*. Minneapolis: CompCare Publishers, 1991.

Huntley, Theresa. *Helping Children Grieve: When Someone They Love Dies*. Minneapolis: Augsburg Fortress, 1991.

Johnson, Kathie J. *Wednesday's Child Is Full of Woe: Helping Children Cope with Grief*. Stockton, Ill.: Hill House, 1991.

Kalina, Kathy. *Midwife for Souls*. Boston: St. Paul Books and Media, 1989.

Kennedy, Alexandra. *Losing a Parent: Passage to a New Way of Living*. San Francisco: HarperSanFrancisco, 1991.

Larson, Hal, and Susan Larson. *Suddenly Single! A Lifeline for Anyone Who Has Lost a Love*. San Francisco: Halo Books, 1990.

Maple, Marilyn. *On the Wings of a Butterfly: A Story About Life and Death*. Seattle: Parenting Press, 1992.

Morgan, John D., ed. *The Dying and the Bereaved Teenager*. Philadelphia: Charles Press, 1990.

O'Toole, Donna. *Aarvy Aardvark Finds Hope*. Burnsville, N.C.: Celo Press, 1988.

Rando, Therese A. *Grieving: How to Go on Living When Someone You Love Dies*. New York: Bantam Books, 1991.

Ray, M. Catherine. *I'm Here to Help*. Mound, Minn.: Hospice Handouts, 1992.

Rosen, Elliot. *Families Facing Death: Family Dynamics of Terminal Illness*. Lexington, Mass.: Lexington Books, 1990.

Sims, Alicia. *Am I Still a Sister?* Wehatchee, Wash.: Big A & Co., 1993.

Smith, Harold. *On Grieving the Death of a Father*. Minneapolis: Augsburg Fortress, 1994.

Tartakoff, Katy. *"My Stupid Illness": The Children's Legacy*. Denver: The Hunt Alternatives Fund, 1991.

Walsh, Froma, and Monica McGoldrick. *Living Beyond Loss: Death in the Family*. New York: Norton, 1991.

SPECIALIZED

Channel 17, WPHL-TV. *Caring for the Frail Elderly: A Resource Guide for the Family*. Philadelphia: WPHL-TV, 1987.

Dane, Barbara O., and Carol Levine, eds. *Aids and the New Orphans: Coping with Death*. Westport, Conn.: Auburn House, 1994.

Fine, Judylaine. *Afraid to Ask: A Book for Families to Share About Cancer*. New York: Lothrop, Lee & Shepard Books, 1986.

Harper, Bernice Catherine. *Death: The Coping Mechanism of the Health Professional*. Greenville, S.C.: Southeastern University Press, 1994.

Jarret, Roberta M. *Caring for the Caregiver: A Nurse's Journey to Health and Inner Peace*. Beaverton, Ore.: Happy Talk Books, 1993.

Kaiser, Charlene, and Hans Van der Giessen. *Home Hospice: A Caregiver's Guide*. Wilton, Conn: Professional Information Consultants, 1988.

National Pediatric HIV Resource Center. *HIV and AIDS in Children — Questions and Answers*.

Rosemire, Adeline. *The Other Mid-Life Crisis: Everything You Need to Know about Wills, Hospitals, Life-and-Death Decisions, and Final Matters (but Were Never Taught)*. San Jose, Calif.: Meridian Publishing Inc., 1994.

Watson, Jeffrey. *The Courage to Care — Helping Aging Grieving and Dying*. Grand Rapids, Mich.: Baker Book House Co., 1992.

Zunin, Leonard M., and Hilary S. *The Art of Condolence: What to Write, What to Say, What to Do at a Time of Loss*. New York: HarperCollins Publishers, 1991.

ACKNOWLEDGMENTS

*T*he concept of hospice is often inspired by a kind of selfless devotion to helping others. The organization of this exhibition and its accompanying book has been motivated by a similar spirit. It would not have been possible to create such a complex document about hospice without a great deal of thoughtful encouragement and the assistance of many people.

We are particularly indebted to the artists, Jim Goldberg, Nan Goldin, Sally Mann, Jack Radcliffe, and Kathy Vargas, who have devoted their time and skills to give us new insights into a difficult subject. We thank them for their courage in accepting the challenge of this arduous commission. Their vision and commitment are evident in this exhibition and book. We are also grateful to Albert Maysles, Susan Froemke, and Deborah Dickson of Maysles Films, Inc., for their enlightening film that accompanies this project. We also must thank our colleague Frances Fralin, whose curatorial contributions in the early stages of this project were critical to the shape it has taken.

The production of this exhibition and book have been complex and multilayered projects. We are indebted to all those people whose professionalism and trust have helped to make them possible. We wish to thank David Levy, Jack Cowart, Susan Badder, Cathy Crane, Paul Roth, Victoria Larson, Ken Ashton, Cindy Rom, Steve Brown, Susan Rosenbaum, John Chappell, Joy Hallinan, Marjory Small, Libby Rogers, Janet Solinger, Suzan Reed, Sher King, George Kimmerling, Shannon Thomas, Erica Weikhardt, and Lisa Chow at the Corcoran Gallery of Art; Zachary Morfogen, John J. Mahoney, Sabrina Allinson, Galen Miller, and Janet Capazo at the National Hospice Foundation and National Hospice Organization; Stuart Lazarus at Learning Design Associates, Inc.; and Sheila Nevins, Jonathan Moss, and Tim Chandler at Home Box Office.

We must give special thanks for the enormous contribution of our publisher, Bulfinch Press, Little, Brown and Company. We are especially grateful to Carol Judy Leslie, publisher, Janet Swan Bush, executive editor, and Terry Reece Hackford, who has skillfully edited the book; and to Caroline Rowntree, who has designed it. Their enthusiasm and faith in this project has been invaluable.

Our appreciation is also extended to Samira K. Beckwith, Ron Culberson, Pat Gibbons, Marcia Lattanzi Licht, Nadine Reimer Penner, Elliot Rosen, Betty Shepperd, Claire Tehan, and Cindy Yocum for their advice on the book's bibliography.

We are also grateful to the staffs of the numerous institutions that will host the exhibition during its national tour, including: Sheri Gelden, Sarah Rogers, Annetta Massie, and Patricia Trumps at the Wexner Center for the Arts; Gregory Knight at the Chicago Cultural Center; Steven Klindt at The Morris Museum; John Buchanan and Terry Toedtemeier at the Portland Art Museum; Steven L. Brezzo at the San Diego Museum of Art; Pamela King at the Telfair Academy of Arts and Sciences; David Stetford at the Norton Gallery and School of Art; Jean Giguet at the Marjorie Barrick Museum of Natural History, University of Nevada, Las Vegas; James K. Ballinger at the Phoenix Art Museum; Diana Johnson at the David Winton Bell Gallery, Brown University; E. John Bullard and Steven Maklansky at the New Orleans Museum of Art; and Patricia McDonnell at the Frederick R. Weisman Art Museum, University of Minnesota, Minneapolis.

Finally, we wish to thank Evelyn Self of Warner-Lambert Company, Kathleen M. Foley, M.D., of the Open Society Institute's Project on Death in America; Dorothy Light of The Prudential Foundation; Betsy Frampton of the Glen Eagles Foundation; and Jennifer Dowley of the National Endowment for the Arts, for their inestimable support of this project.

Dena Andre, Philip Brookman, and Jane Livingston

PHOTOGRAPHERS' ACKNOWLEDGMENTS

Jim Goldberg

I would like to thank all the people who have given me their guidance, friendship, and time during my work on this project. I am most grateful to Fran A. Brunell and the rest of the Hospice of the Florida Suncoast Green Team: Cosette Freeman, Joan Lauzon, Fran Nelson, Ray Sunter, Darryl Thompson, Estelle Thurm, and Carol Wolf. I also wish to acknowledge the support of Patricia Murphy of the Visiting Nurses and Hospice of San Francisco, Larry Beresford, Ed Lorah, and Adam. I am especially grateful to Lorelei Stewart and to James Dawson, Hannah Frost, and Tony Tredway for their continued assistance. I wish to give special thanks to my collaborators — Lillian Goldberg, the Goldberg family, the Kormans — and above all to Susan, Ruby, and Herb.

Nan Goldin

I would most of all like to thank my assistant Jenna Ward, who came with me on each hospice visit. It was important for me to go through these experiences with someone from my own life whom I could share them with. She became deeply involved in her own relationships with the hospice patients and continued visiting them when I was out of town. Thanks also to: Rick Colon; Debbie Sior, assistant to executive director, Priscilla Ruffin, executive director, and volunteer Robert Trepeta from East End Hospice; Paul Brenner, director, Jacob Perlow Hospice, Beth Israel Medical Center; and especially Mary Cooke and her staff at Cabrini Hospice; and to all the people who allowed me to photograph them.

Sally Mann

Obviously, this project would not have been possible without Joan Robins. I am thankful for her patience and good humor in helping me, as well as for the dedication, sensitivity, and respect with which she treats her patients. She is a rare and generous friend.

I am grateful to the Rockbridge Area Hospice for its support of this project. I especially would like to thank Susan Hogg, Lisa Hinty, Nell Bolen, Amy Hefty, Karen Hostetter, Debbie Barron, and Karen Agura.

I appreciate the trust that the families showed in letting me come into their lives at such a difficult time. As always, I am grateful to my own family for allowing me to take on another intensive project. I'm especially indebted to Betsy Schneider and Katie Kirtland. Finally, Niall MacKenzie, as you know, this is yours.

Jack Radcliffe

I wish to express my heartfelt thanks to Barbara Ellen Wood, who has worked with me since my first visit to York House Hospice and has faithfully kept a diligent record of our experiences. My admiration goes to Joy Ufema, a person of heroic stature, whose spirituality, devotion to the concept of hospice, and singleminded commitment to the patients' minds as well as their bodies are the heart and soul of York House. I also extend my admiration to the staff of York House, who under Joy's leadership, perform with similar dedication. I express my very high regard for Dr. David Hawk, who has always displayed kindness and warmth for each patient. And finally I wish to acknowledge my special gratitude to those I photographed, and their families and friends, who opened their lives to me with the hope that York House would benefit from their candor and continue to be there for future patients.

Kathy Vargas

Special thanks to: Don Bacigalupi; Stacy Zacharias; Penelope Alice Boyer, Donald Day Boyer, Katherine Eleanor Boyer Reisert, and the entire Boyer family; Sharen Rupp of the San Antonio AIDS Foundation, Robert Rupp, and Pat Day of Santa Rosa Hospice; Dr. Marion P. Primomo of Family Hospice of San Antonio and Richard Smith; Jason Piercy, Brandon Haga, and Cindy Lengel of Project Transitions, Austin, Texas, and Woody; Jack and Vivian Yatteau; Helen Gardner and Ruth Landauer of The Hospice at the Texas Medical Center, Houston, Texas, and Jaime Gerson; Millie DeAnda, Fred Hines, and Sue Dial of Hospice San Antonio, and Lisa and Lauren Saegert.

Biography: JIM GOLDBERG

Born   New Haven, Connecticut, June 3, 1953
Education   Western Washington University, Bellingham, Washington,
                BA, 1975
                San Francisco Art Institute, San Francisco, California, MFA, 1979
                Lives and works in San Francisco, California

Selected Solo Exhibitions

1995   "Raised by Wolves," organized by the Corcoran Gallery of Art,
        Washington, D.C., and Addison Gallery of American Art,
        Andover, Massachusetts (traveling exhibition/catalogue)
1991   Art in General, New York City
1990   Washington Project for the Arts, Washington, D.C.
        "Art at the Anchorage," Creative Time, New York City
1989   Capp Street Project, San Francisco, California
1988   Washington Project for the Arts, Washington, D.C.
        Museum of Photographic Arts, San Diego, California
1987   Akron Art Museum, Akron, Ohio
        Clarence Kennedy Gallery, Cambridge, Massachusetts
        University Art Museum, Berkeley, California
1986   The Tartt Gallery, Washington, D.C.
1985   Northlight Gallery, Tempe, Arizona
        Ithaca College, Ithaca, New York
        De Saisset Museum, Santa Clara, California
        G. H. Dalsheimer Gallery, Baltimore, Maryland
1984   Houston Center for Photography, Houston, Texas
        Indiana University, Bloomington, Indiana
        Friends of Photography Gallery, Carmel, California
        Lightsong Gallery, Tucson, Arizona
1982   Blue Sky Gallery, Portland, Oregon
1981   O. K. Harris Gallery, New York City
1980   Equivalents Gallery, Seattle, Washington
1979   Nova Gallery, Vancouver, B.C., Canada

Selected Group Exhibitions

1994   "Who's Looking at the Family?" Barbican Art Gallery,
        London (catalogue)
1990   "IV Fotobienal — 90" Vigo, Spain (catalogue)
        "Rethinking American Myths," Laurence Miller Gallery,
        New York City (traveling exhibition)
1988   "Recent Acquisitions," National Museum of American Art,
        Washington, D.C.
        "Collecting on the Cutting Edge: Frito-Lay, Inc.," Laguna
        Gloria Art Museum, Austin, Texas
        "The Instant Likeness: Polaroid Portraits," National Portrait
        Gallery, Washington, D.C.
1987   "Legacy of Light: Polaroid Photographs by 58 Photographers"
        (traveling exhibition/catalogue)
        "Mothers & Daughters," Burden Gallery, Aperture
        Foundation, New York City (traveling exhibition/catalogue)
1985   "Extending the Perimeters of 20th Century Photography,"
        San Francisco Museum of Modern Art, San Francisco,
        California (catalogue)
1984   "Three Americans (Robert Adams, Joel Sternfeld, Jim
        Goldberg), Museum of Modern Art, New York City
        "Photography in California: 1945–1980," San Francisco
        Museum of Modern Art, San Francisco, California
        (catalogue)
1983   "20th Century Photographs from the Museum of Modern
        Art, New York," Seibu Museum of Art, Tokyo
        (catalogue)
        "Bay Area Collects," San Francisco Museum of Modern
        Art, San Francisco, California
1980   "Ruth Bernhard and Jim Goldberg," Equivalents Gallery,
        Seattle, Washington

"Form, Freud, and Feeling," San Francisco Museum of
        Modern Art, San Francisco, California
1979   "Exploring the Documentary," Mary Porter Sesnon Gallery,
        University of California, Santa Cruz, California
        "Photographs," San Francisco Museum of Modern Art, San
        Francisco, California (catalogue)
        "Voice and Vision: Photographs of Jim Goldberg, Duane
        Michaels, Harvey Stein, and James Van Der Zee,"
        Creative Photography Gallery, Cambridge, Massachusetts

Selected Grants, Fellowships, and Awards

Documentary Book of the Year, Maine Photographic Workshop, 1995
Roberts Foundation Grant, 1995
Highland Award, 1994
Glen Eagles Foundation Grant, 1992
Art Matters, Inc., New York, 1989, 1992
Fellowship in Photography, National Endowment for the Arts, 1980, 1989,
        1990
California Arts Council Fellowship, 1990
Jaffe Award, 1989
T. B. Walker Foundation, 1989
California Tamarack Foundation, 1989
John Simon Guggenheim Memorial Foundation Fellowship, 1985
Engelhard Award, Boston, Massachusetts, 1985
Cambridge Art Council Commission, 1985
Ruttenberg Fellowship, 1983

Books by Jim Goldberg

Raised by Wolves. Zurich: Scalo, 1995.
Rich and Poor. New York: Random House, 1985.

Selected Bibliography

Atkins, Robert. "Letters," *Contemporanea*, No. 22 (November 1990): 30.
Fallon, D'Arcy. "Faces From the Streets," *San Francisco Examiner*, 8 May 1989,
        B1–3.
Green, J. Ronald. "After Agee," *Aperture*, No. 112 (fall 1988): 72–77.
Grundberg, Andy. "The New Modern Re-enters the Contemporary Arena,"
        New York Times, 27 May 1984.
————. "A New Era of Image-Making," *New York Times*, 30 December 1985.
Harper, Hilliard. "Invisible People Exhibit Pierces the Soul," *Los Angeles
        Times*, 18 March 1988.
Indiana, Gary. "Home," *Aperture* (spring 1992): 56–63.
Muchnic, Suzanne. "Two Exhibitions That Show and Tell," *Los Angeles Times*,
        18 February 1986, 5.
Smith, Roberta. "In a Show on the Issues, the Focus is Outrage." *New York
        Times*, 27 July 1990.
Stapen, Nancy. "Cambridge, MA, Jim Goldberg," *Artforum* (summer 1987):
        123.
Starenko, Michael. "Words and Pictures — Three Americans: Photographs by
        Robert Adams, Jim Goldberg, and Joel Sternfeld," *Afterimage* (October
        1984): 14–15.
Steinman, Louise. "Endangered Species: Jim Goldberg's Work in Progress, Capp
        Street Project," *Artscribe* (September/October 1989).
Strauss, David Levi. "The Youngest Homeless: A Threnody for Street Kids,"
        The Nation (June 1, 1992): 752–54.
Weber, John. "Narrative in North America," *European Photography*, No. 24
        (December 1985): 16.
Westerbeck, Colin. "Rich and Poor," *Exposure* (summer 1986): 45.
Wise, Kelly. "Jim Goldberg," *All Things Considered*, National Public Radio
        (February 1987).
————. "Images of Rich and Poor in Black and White," *Boston Globe*, 13
        December 1986.
Wollheim, Peter. "Cumming/Goldberg/Woodman, Beyond Semiotics," *Photo-
        Communique* (summer 1987): 9.

Biography: NAN GOLDIN

Born   Washington, D.C., September 12, 1953
Education   Imageworks, Cambridge, Massachusetts, 1974
             School of the Museum of Fine Arts/Tufts University, Boston,
               Massachusetts, BA/BFA, 1977
             Lives and works in New York City

Selected Solo Exhibitions

1995   Centre d'Art Contemporain, Geneva, Switzerland
        Matthew Marks Gallery, New York City
        Rebecca Camhi Gallery, Athens, Greece
        Galerie Yvon Lambert, Paris, France
1994   Jeffrey Fraenkel Gallery, San Francisco, California
        Bruno Brunnet Fine Arts, Berlin, Germany
        Nationalgalerie, Berlin, Germany
        "Tokyo Love," Shiscido Artspace, Tokyo, Japan
1993   Matthew Marks Gallery, New York City
        Pace/MacGill Gallery, New York City
        "La Vida Sin Amor No Tiene Sentido," Fundacio La Caixa,
          Barcelona, Spain
        Fotografiska Museet, Moderna Museet, Stockholm, Sweden
1992   Galerie M, Bochum, Germany
        DAAD Galerie, Berlin, Germany
        "Obsessions," Orangerie, Münich, Germany
1991   Folkwang Museum, Essen, Germany
        PPS Galerie, Hamburg, Germany
        Galerie Urbi et Orbi, Paris, France
        Forum Stadtpark, Graz, Austria
        Shoshana Wayne Gallery, Santa Monica, California
1990   Pace/MacGill Gallery, New York City
1988   "Couples," Pace/MacGill Gallery, New York City
1987   Les Rencontres d'Arles, Arles, France
        Middendorf Gallery, Washington, D. C.
1986   Burden Gallery, Aperture Foundation, New York City
1985   "Currents," Institute of Contemporary Art, Boston,
          Massachusetts
1973   Project, Inc., Cambridge, Massachusetts

Selected Group Exhibitions

1995   "Biennial Exhibition," Whitney Museum of American Art,
          New York City
        "Public Information: Desire, Disaster, Document," San
          Francisco Museum of Modern Art, San Francisco,
          California
1994   "Welt Moral," Kunsthalle, Basel, Switzerland
1993   "Biennial Exhibition," Whitney Museum of American Art,
          New York City
        "Bad Girls," Institute of Contemporary Art, London, U.K.
1992   "Desordres," Jeu de Paume, Paris, France
1991   "Devil on the Stairs: Looking Back on the '80's," Institute of
          Contemporary Art, Philadelphia, Pennsylvania
        "Pleasures and Terrors of Domestic Comfort," Museum of
          Modern Art, New York City
1988   "Real Faces," Whitney Museum of American Art, Philip
          Morris Branch, New York City
1985   "Biennial Exhibition," Whitney Museum of American Art,
          New York City

Selected Grants, Fellowships, and Awards

Emery Award, Hetrick-Martin Institute, New York City, 1994
Brandeis Award in Photography, Brandeis University, Waltham, Massachusetts,
   1994
Golden Light Photographic Book of the Year Award, Maine Photographic
   Workshop, 1993
Louis Comfort Tiffany Foundation Award, 1991
DAAD, Artists-in-Residence Program, Berlin, Germany, 1991
National Endowment for the Arts, 1990
Mother Jones Documentary Photography Award, San Francisco, California,
   1990
Art Matters, Inc., New York, 1990
Camera Austria Prize for Contemporary Photography, Graz, Austria, 1989
Documentary Book of the Year, Maine Photographic Workshop, 1987
Photographic Book Prize of the Year, Les Rencontres d'Arles, France, 1987
Kodak Photoduchpreis, Stuttgart, Germany, 1987
Englehard Award, Boston, Massachusetts, 1986
School of the Museum of Fine Arts Alumni Traveling Fellowship, Boston,
   Massachusetts, 1986
Clarissa Bartlett Traveling Fellowship, Boston, Massachusetts, 1978
Wilhelmina Jackson Fellowship, Marblehead, Massachusetts, 1977

Books by Nan Goldin

The Ballad of Sexual Dependency. New York: Aperture, 1986 (German edition
   published by 2001, Germany, 1986; British edition published by Secker &
   Warburg, London, 1989).
Cookie Mueller. New York: Pace/MacGill Gallery, 1991.
Desire by Numbers. San Francisco: Artspace, 1994, with text by Klaus Kertess.
A Double Life. Zurich: Scalo, 1994, with David Armstrong.
The Other Side. Zurich: Scalo, 1992. (Japanese edition published by Déjà Vu,
   1993).
Tokyo Love. Tokyo: Hon Hon Do, 1994, with Nobuyoshi Araki.
Vakat. Köln: Walther Konig, 1993, with poems by Joachim Sartorius.

Selected Bibliography

Als, Hilton. "The Third Set," *Artforum* (January 1994): 58–63.
Bracewell, Michael. "Making Up Is Hard to Do," *Frieze* (September/October
   1993): 32–37.
De Lombard, Jeannine. "The Posed and the Exposed," *New York Times Book
   Review,* 8 August 1993, 20.
Dicckmann, Katherine. "Back from the Brink," *Village Voice,* 18 September
   1990.
———. "Queen's Logic," *Village Voice,* 18 May 1993.
Friis-Hansen, Dana. "Nan Goldin/Nobuyoshi Araki," *Flash Art* (January/
   February 1995): 108.
Grossfeld, Stan. "Philip-Lorca DiCorciaf's Reputation Outruns His Work,"
   Boston Globe, 25 December 1993, 40.
Grundberg, Andy. "So, What Else Do You Want to Know About Me?" *New
   York Times,* 21 September 1990.
Hagen, Charles. "A Monumental Slide Show at a New Gallery," *New York
   Times,* 10 February 1995, C24.
Hess, Elizabeth. "The Family of Nan," *Village Voice,* 18 May 1993.
Holborn, Mark. "Nan Goldin's Ballad of Sexual Dependency," *Aperture,* No.
   103 (summer 1986): 38–47.
Howell, John. "Books: A Review of David Byrne and Nan Goldin," *Artforum*
   (October 1986): 8–10.
Kozloff, Max. "The Family of Nan," *Art in America* (November 1987): 38–43.
Schjeldahl, Peter. "One-Man Show: Klauss Kertess's Biennial *Moyen Sensuel,*"
   Village Voice, 4 April 1995, 72–73.
———. "The Goldin Age," *Vogue* (March 1995): 394–97, 458.
Westfall, Stephen. "The Ballad of Nan Goldin," *Bomb* (fall 1991).
Wise, Kelly. "Engaging Images of Illusion and Irony," *Boston Globe,* 20 May
   1991, 45.

Biography: SALLY MANN

Born Lexington, Virginia, May 1, 1951
Education Putney School, Bennington College and Friends World
College, Bennington, Vermont, 1966–72
Hollins College, Roanoke, Virginia, BA (*summa cum laude*),
1974
Hollins College, Roanoke, Virginia, MA, 1975
Lives and works in Lexington, Virginia

Selected Solo Exhibitions
1995 "Sally Mann: Recent Work," Houk Friedman, New York City
"Sally Mann: At Twelve and Color Work," Picture Photo
Space, Osaka, Japan
1994 "Selections from *Immediate Family,*" Bratislava, Slovakia
"Immediate Family," The Contemporary Museum, Honolulu,
Hawaii
1993 "Still Time," Museum of Contemporary Photography,
Chicago, Illinois (traveling exhibition)
"Selections from *Immediate Family,*" The Center for Creative
Photography, Carmel, California
"Selections from *Immediate Family,*" Photo Gallery
International, Tokyo, Japan
1992 "Immediate Family," Houk Friedman, New York City
"Immediate Family," Institute of Contemporary Art,
Philadelphia, Pennsylvania
"At Twelve," Edwynn Houk Gallery, Chicago, Illinois
1991 Maryland Art Place, Baltimore, Maryland
1990 The Tartt Gallery, Washington, D.C.
Edwynn Houk Gallery, Chicago, Illinois
Cleveland Center for Contemporary Art, Cleveland, Ohio
1989 Museum of Photographic Arts, San Diego, California
1988 Marcuse Pfeiffer Gallery, New York City
Southeastern Center for Contemporary Art, Winston-Salem,
North Carolina
"Sally Mann: Still Time," Allegheny Highlands Arts and
Crafts Center, Clifton Forge, Virginia (catalogue)
1987 "Sally Mann: Sweet Silent Thought," North Carolina Center
for Creative Photography, Durham, North Carolina
1977 "The Lewis Law Portfolio," the Corcoran Gallery of Art,
Washington, D.C. (catalogue)

Selected Group Exhibitions
1995 "100 Years/100 Images," Frankfurter Kunstverein, Frankfurt,
Germany
"Visions of Childhood," Bard College, Annandale-on-
Hudson, New York
1994 "Who's Looking at the Family?" Barbican Art Gallery,
London, U.K.
"Profemina," Southeast Museum of Photography, Daytona
Beach, Florida
1993 "Elegant Intimacy," The Retretti Museum, Finland
"Prospect 93," Frankfurter Kunstverein and the Schirn
Kunsthalle, Frankfurt, Germany
1991 "Pleasures and Terrors of Domestic Comfort," Museum of
Modern Art, New York City
"The Body in Question," Burden Gallery, Aperture
Foundation, New York City
"Biennial Exhibition," Whitney Museum of American Art,
New York City
1990 "Awards in the Visual Arts 9," New Orleans Museum of Art,
New Orleans, Louisiana (traveling exhibition)
1988 "Un/Common Ground," Virginia Museum, Richmond,
Virginia (catalogue)
1987 "Mothers & Daughters," Burden Gallery, Aperture Founda-
tion, New York City (traveling exhibition/catalogue)

"Legacy of Light: Polaroid Photographs by 58 Photographers"
(traveling exhibition/catalogue)
1985 "Big Shots: 20 x 24 Polaroid Photographs," Visual Arts
Gallery, University of Alabama, Birmingham, Alabama
(traveling exhibition/catalogue)
1982 "The Ferguson Grant Winners Show," Friends of
Photography, Carmel, California
1980 "Not Fade Away: Four Contemporary Virginia
Photographers," The Chrysler Museum, Norfolk, Virginia

Selected Grants, Fellowships, and Awards
"Photographer of the Year" Award, Friends of Photography, 1995
National Endowment for the Arts, 1982, 1988, 1992
Artists in the Visual Arts Fellowship (AVA), 1989
SECCA Artists Fellowship, 1989
John Simon Guggenheim Memorial Foundation Fellowship, 1987
Virginia Museum of Fine Arts Professional Fellowship, 1982
Ferguson Grant, Friends of Photography, 1974
National Endowment for the Humanities, 1973, 1976

Books by Sally Mann
At Twelve: Portraits of Young Women. New York: Aperture Foundation, Inc., 1988.
Immediate Family. New York: Aperture Foundation, Inc., 1992.
Second Sight: The Photographs of Sally Mann. Boston: David Godine Publisher, 1982.
Still Time. New York: Aperture Foundation, Inc., 1994.

Selected Bibliography
Aukeman, A. *Art in America* (February 1992): 23.
Balz, Douglas. "Controversial Intimacies," *Chicago Tribune*, 6 December 1992,
sec. 14, p. 3.
Christensen, J. "A Sense of Place," *Artweek* (April 22, 1989): 11–12.
Coleman, A. D. "New York, No. 36: Sally Mann and Jock Sturges," in *Critical
Focus* (Munich: Nazraeli Press, 1995), pp. 146–55.
Douglas, A. "Blood Ties," *Women's Art Magazine* (1994): 20–21.
Ellenzweig, A. *Art in America* (January 1987): 140.
Eugenides, Jeffrey. "Sally Mann: Jeffrey Hayhook, 1989," *Artforum* (December
1994): 56–57.
Foerstner, Abigail. "Sally Mann Records 12-Year-Olds' Changing World,"
Chicago Tribune, 22 May 1992, sec. 7, p. 89.
———. "The Family of Mann," *Chicago Tribune*, 19 September 1993, sec. 13,
p. 30.
Hagen, Charles. "Childhood Without Sweetness," *New York Times*, 5 June 1992.
Harris, M. "Truths Told Slant," *Artforum* (summer 1992): 102–04.
Jenkins, S. "Motherly Love," *Artweek* (June 3, 1993): 19.
Jones, P. C. "Hot Photographers," *Connoisseur* (November 1990): 150–52.
Liu, C. "In the Realm of the Senses," *Flash Art* (October 1988): 100–01.
Malcolm, Janet. "The Family of Mann," *New York Review of Books*, 3 February
1994.
Morgan, R. C. *Arts Magazine* (December 1988): 102.
Price, R. "Neighbors and Kin: Four Southern Photographers," *Aperture* (sum-
mer 1989): 32–39.
Orland, T. "Traces of Memory," *Artweek* (November 6, 1982): 11.
Sante, Luc. "The Nude and the Naked," *New Republic* (May 1, 1995): 30.
Schonauer, D., et al. "Photography's Top 100," *American Photo*
(January/February 1994): 94.
Schwendenwien, J. *New Art Examiner* (April 1993): 35.
Shepherd, Rose. "Sally Mann," *London Times Sunday Magazine*, 22 May 1994.
Shimon, J., and J. Lindemann, "Blood Relatives: The Family in Contemporary
Photography," *New Art Examiner* (September 1991): 41–42.
Williams, V. "Fragile Innocence: Issues Raised When Intimate Family
Photographs Become Public," *British Journal of Photography* (October 15,
1992): 10.
Woodward, Richard. "The Disturbing Photography of Sally Mann," *New York
Times Magazine*, 27 September 1992, sec. 6, p. 29.

Biography: JACK RADCLIFFE

Born Elizabeth, New Jersey, September 17, 1940
Education Grove City College, Grove City, Pennsylvania, BA, 1963
University of Maryland, College Park, Maryland, MA, 1970
Lives and works in Baltimore, Maryland

Selected Solo Exhibitions

1993 "Work in Progress: Photography by Jack Radcliffe," College
of Notre Dame of Maryland, Baltimore, Maryland
Nye Gomez Gallery, Baltimore, Maryland
1988 Knight Gomez Gallery, Baltimore, Maryland
Northern Virginia Community College, Alexandria, Virginia
1986 G. H. Dalsheimer Gallery, Baltimore, Maryland

Selected Group Exhibitions

1993 "Proof Positive," The Maryland Art Place, Baltimore,
Maryland (brochure)
"Photo Review," Hemicycle Gallery, the Corcoran Gallery of
Art, Washington, D.C.
1992 "The American Dream," Woodstock Center for Photography,
Woodstock, New York
"Photowork '92," Coral Gables, Florida
1991 Toledo Friends of Photography, Toledo, Ohio
Washington Center for Photography, Washington, D.C.
Woodstock Center for Photography, Woodstock, New York
1989 "Recent Acquisitions," the Corcoran Gallery of Art,
Washington, D.C.
"Maryland Invitational," Baltimore Museum of Art,
Baltimore, Maryland
1988 "Jack Radcliffe and Connie Imboden," Goucher College,
Towson, Maryland
"Artscape '88," Baltimore, Maryland
1987 "Mothers & Daughters," Burden Gallery, Aperture
Foundation, New York City (traveling exhibition/
catalogue)
1985 "Contemporary American Photographers," Baltimore
Museum of Art, Baltimore, Maryland
1984 Goucher College, Towson, Maryland
1983 Foundry Gallery, Washington, D.C.
"Artscape '83," Baltimore, Maryland
1982 "Washington Photography: Images of the Eighties," the
Corcoran Gallery of Art, Washington, D.C. (traveling
exhibition/catalogue)
"Nine Photographers," Goucher College, Towson, Maryland
1981 "Recent Acquisitions," the Corcoran Gallery of Art,
Washington, D.C.

Selected Grants, Fellowships, and Awards

Baltimore City Arts Grant, 1992
Maryland State Arts Council, 1991
Baltimore City Arts Grant, 1991
Maryland State Arts Council, 1988
Maryland State Arts Council, 1985

Selected Bibliography

Cerquone, Joseph. "Capturing the Human Connection," *Hospice* (fall 1994).
Dorsey, John. "Evocative Photographs Delve Beneath the Surface," *Baltimore Sun,* 23 September 1988.
———. "A New Gallery in South Baltimore Will Take Chances," *Baltimore Sun,* 15 December 1988.
———. "Loss of Catalogue and Tour Mar Otherwise Improved Maryland Invitational," *Baltimore Sun,* 27 February 1989, sec. 1B.
———. "Proof Positive Captures a Good Life Despite HIV," *Baltimore Sun,* 11 December 1993, sec. 5D.
Durantine, Peter. "Different Drums Beat Together on United Day," *York Daily Record,* 28 June 1993.
Fleming, Lee. "Washington Photography: Striking Views," *Washingtonian Magazine* (April 1982): 55.
Giuliano, Mike. "Select Artists Blend Well at the BMA," *Columbia Flyer,* 9 March 1989.
Kimmel, Carolyn Jenko. "These Are Not Ogres: Local Images Are in National Hospice Display," *York Dispatch,* 25 October 1994.
MacGill, Peter. "Review," *Toledo Friends of Photography Newsletter* (November 1991).
Perloff, Stephen. "The 1991 Photo Review Competition Winners," *Photo Review* (summer 1991): 20.
———. "The 1993 Photo Review Competition Winners," *Photo Review* (summer 1993).
———. "Jack Radcliffe," *Photo Review Newsletter* (August/September 1993).
Purchase, Steve. "Photos of Mixed Emotions," *Evening Sun,* 27 September 1988.
Richard, Paul. "The Power of the Picture: 11 Photographers at the Corcoran & Beauty's Intriguing Complexity," *Washington Post,* 20 February 1982, sec. C1, p. 20.
Scarupa, Henry. "Artists Chosen for Invitational," *Baltimore Sun,* 6 February 1988.
Toussaint, Karen. "Tenderness with an Edge," *Aegis,* 3 June 1992.
Wittenberg, Clarissa. "Washington Photography: Images of the Eighties," *Washington Review* (April/May 1982): 29–30.
"Photographs by Connie Imboden and John [sic] Radcliffe," *Citypaper,* 6 September 1988.
"Portfolio: Jack Radcliffe," *American Arts Magazine* (September 1983).

Biography: KATHY VARGAS

Born San Antonio, Texas, June 23, 1950
Education University of Texas at San Antonio, BFA, 1981
University of Texas at San Antonio, MFA, 1984
Lives and works in San Antonio, Texas

Selected Solo Exhibitions

1994 Lynn Good Gallery, Houston, Texas
Jump Start Performance Space, San Antonio, Texas
1993 "Images of Loss and Hope," Houston Center for
Photography, Houston, Texas (traveling exhibition)
Galerie Posada, Sacramento, California
1992 Jansen-Perez Gallery, San Antonio, Texas
1991 Louisiana State University, Shreveport, Louisiana
University of Texas at El Paso, El Paso, Texas
1990 "Kathy Vargas: Priests Series and Oracion: Valentine's
Day/Day of the Dead Series," Frances Wolfson Art
Gallery, Miami Dade Community College, Miami, Florida
(catalogue)
1989 Pinnacle Gallery, Dallas, Texas
1988 Universitat Erlangen-Nurnberg, Erlangen, Germany
San Angelo Museum of Fine Art, San Angelo, Texas
1987 Biblioteca Simon Bolivar; Centro de Ensenanza para
Extranjeros, Universidad Nacional Autonoma de Mexico,
Mexico City, Mexico
1986 Galerie Fotocamera, Grosseto, Italy
1985 Women's Center, University of California, Santa Barbara,
California
1984 Galleria Sala Uno, Rome, Italy
Galeria Juan Martin, Mexico City, Mexico
Amerika Haus, Stuttgart, Germany
Charlton Gallery, San Antonio, Texas

Selected Group Exhibitions

1995 "The Pleasure Principle," CEPA Gallery, Buffalo, New York
1994 "American Photography: A History in Pictures," San
Antonio Museum of Art, San Antonio, Texas
1993 "Target: South Texas — Depth of Field," Art Museum of
South Texas, Corpus Christi, Texas (catalogue)
1992 "From Media to Metaphor: Art about AIDS," Emerson
Gallery, Hamilton College, Clinton, New York (traveling
exhibition/catalogue)
"The Chicano Codices: Encountering Art of the Americas,"
Mexican Museum, San Francisco, California (traveling
exhibition/catalogue)
1991 "Oraciones Para los Desasesinados" with Diana Cardenas,
Women & Their Work, Austin, Texas
"Contemporary Hispanic Women Artists of Texas,"
The Art Center, Waco, Texas (traveling exhibition/
catalogue)
1990 "Mixing It Up," University of Colorado, Boulder, Colorado
"Emulsionally Involved," Images Gallery, Cincinnati, Ohio
"Chicano Art: Resistance and Affirmation," Wight Art
Gallery, University of California, Los Angeles, California
(traveling exhibition/catalogue)
1988 "The Presence of the Sublime," San Antonio Museum of
Art, San Antonio, Texas (traveling exhibition/catalogue)
1987 "Third Coast Review: A Look at Art in Texas," Aspen Art
Museum, Aspen, Colorado (traveling exhibition/
catalogue)
"Spaces in the Heart of Texas," Women & Their Work,
Austin, Texas
1985 "Fotografica: Las Americas — Toward A New Perspective,"
Gallery 1199, New York City (traveling exhibition)

1984 "Texas Women Photographers Today," Canon Photo
Gallery, Amsterdam, The Netherlands
"Tercer Coloquio Latinoamericano de Fotografia," Casa de
las Americas, Havana, Cuba
1981 "Hecho en Latinoamerica II," Bellas Artes, Mexico City,
Mexico

Selected Grants, Fellowships, and Awards

Pace-Roberts Foundation Residency, 1995
Mid-American Arts Alliance Grant (regional)/National Endowment for the
Arts, 1995
Individual Artist's Grant, Department of Arts and Cultural Affairs, City of
San Antonio, 1991

Selected Bibliography

Bruce-Novoa, Juan. "El Arte de Kathryn Vargas," *La Opinion*, 23 October,
1983, *La Comunidad Sunday Supplement*, 4–6.
Goddard, Dan R. "San Antonio/Kathy Vargas/Jansen Perez Gallery," *Latin
American Art* (winter 1992): 92–93 (English), 117–118 (Spanish).
Goldman, Saundra. "Contemporary Hispanic Women Artists," *Art Papers*
(September/October 1991): 61–62.
Goldman, Shifra. "Artistas Chicanas Texanas," *fem.* (June/July 1984): 29–31.
———. "Kathy Vargas," *Nueva Luz, A Photographic Journal* 4, No.2, (1993):
2–11, 32–33, cover.
Highberg, Nels P. "Postcards from the Edge," *SPOT* (spring 1993): 19.
Hulick, Diana Emery. "Immortalizing Death — The Photography of Kathy
Vargas," *Latin American Art* (fall 1994): 62–65.
Johnson, Patricia C. "Putting on Happy Front," *Houston Chronicle*, 26 August
1991, sec. D, pp. 1, 6.
Johnson, Richard. "Chicano Images Live On," *Denver Post*, 20 January 1993,
sec. F, pp. 1, 3.
Lineberrry, Heather Sealy. "Post-Chicano Art at MARS," *The Art Link
Letter* 1 (winter 1990): 1.
Lippard, Lucy. *Mixed Blessings: New Art in a Multicultural America* (New York:
Pantheon Books, 1990), pp. 84–85.
———. *The Pink Glass Swan* (New York: The New Press, 1995), p. 206.
Perrone, Jeff. "Point of No Return," *Arts Magazine* (December 1985): 89.
Robinson, Joan Seeman. "Contra-Positions," *SPOT* (summer 1988): 14–15.
Torres, Alma Isabel. "Exhibiran aqui una probadita de arte chicano," *El Norte*,
13 June 1992, sec. D5.
Tyson, Janet. "Artists Explore Topic of Death," *Fort Worth Star-Telegram*,
January 1991.
Weser, Marcia Goren. "Vargas Finds Multiple Meanings," *San Antonio Light*,
25 October 1992, sec. J5.